SCORE SERIOUS RESULTS

KETO FOR CARB LOVERS

AND EAT FOODS YOU LOVE!

100+
AMAZING LOW-CARB, HIGH-FAT RECIPES!

FROM THE EDITORS OF delish & Women's Health

This book is intended as a reference volume only, not as a medical manual. The information given here is designed to help you make informed decisions about your health. It is not intended as a substitute for any treatment that may have been prescribed by your doctor. If you suspect that you have a medical problem, we urge you to seek competent medical help.

Mention of specific companies, organizations, or authorities in this book does not imply endorsement by the author or publisher, nor does mention of specific companies, organizations, or authorities imply that they endorse this book, its author, or the publisher.

Internet addresses and phone numbers given in this book were accurate at the time it went to press.

© 2020 by Hearst Magazines, Inc.

All rights reserved. No part of this publication may be reproduced or transmitted in any form or by any means, electronic or mechanical, including photocopying, recording, or any other information storage and retrieval system, without the written permission of the publisher.

Printed in China

Photographs by Parker Feierbach and Emily Hlavic Green
Book Design by Lauren Vitello

Library of Congress Cataloging-in-Publication Data
is on file with the publisher.

978-1-950099-45-0
12 paperback

HEARST

TABLE OF CONTENTS

EVERYTHING YOU NEED TO KNOW ABOUT KETO 8
- *The Secret to Satisfying Your Carb Cravings* 8
- *How to Ditch Carbs and Feel Like You're Eating Them, Too* 8
- *7 Reasons You'll Love The Keto Diet* 9
- *Your Keto Questions, Answered* 10
- *The 3 Rules of Keto for Carb Lovers* 11
- *How to Ace Week 1* 11
- *7 Keto-Approved Foods and Snacks for Carb Lovers* 12

HOW TO FOLLOW THE 21-DAY PLAN 14

#BREAKFASTGOALS 32
- *Cauliflower Toast* 33
- *Pizza Eggs* 33
- *Bunless Bacon, Egg & Cheese* 34
- *Avocado Egg-In-A-Hole* 35
- *Perfect Pancakes* 37
- *Baked Egg Avocado Boats* 38
- *Breakfast Wraps* 39
- *Taco Brunch Casserole* 41
- *Ham & Cheese Egg Cups* 42
- *Loaded Cauliflower Breakfast Bake* 44
- *Ham, Egg & Cheese Roll-Ups* 45
- *Everything Keto Bagels* 47
- *Bacon Weave Breakfast Tacos* 48
- *Cauli Breakfast Hash* 50

POWER LUNCHES — 52
- Zucchini Grilled Cheese — 53
- Spicy Chicken Sandwich — 54
- Taco Cups — 57
- Cobb Egg Salad — 58
- Ta-Ketos — 61
- Low-Carb Garlic Bread Dogs — 62
- No-Bread Italian Subs — 63
- Turkey Club Cups — 63
- Fat Head Supreme Pizza — 64
- BLT Burgers — 66
- Chicken Parm Pizza — 67
- Cheeseburger Cabbage Wraps — 69

LOW-CARB COMFORT FOODS — 70
- Loaded Cheese Taco Shells — 71
- No-Carb Philly Cheesesteaks — 72
- Cheesy Lasagna — 75
- Slow-Cooked Beef Stroganoff — 76
- Egg Roll Bowls — 79
- Bacon-Wrapped Meatloaf — 80
- Pizza-Stuffed Zucchini — 83
- Biscuits & Gravy — 84
- Zoodle Alfredo with Bacon — 87
- Garlic Rosemary Pork Chops — 88
- Mac & Cheese — 91
- Cauliflower Baked Ziti — 92
- Chicken Piccata — 94
- Crispy Chicken & Waffles — 97
- Jalapeño Popper Chicken Casserole — 98
- Antipasto Stuffed Chicken — 101
- Creamy Tuscan Chicken — 102

INSANELY EASY SEAFOOD & VEGGIES — 104

Chilean Sea Bass with Spinach-Avocado Pesto — 105
Best Greek Salad — 106
Tuscan Butter Salmon — 109
Avocado Crab Boats — 110
Breaded Shrimp — 111
Rosemary-Dijon Salmon — 112
Bruschetta Swordfish — 115
Grilled Salmon & Lemony Asparagus Foil Packs — 116
Spinach-Artichoke Stuffed Mushrooms — 118
Creamed Spinach Stuffed Salmon — 119
Garlicky Lemon Mahi-Mahi — 121
Lemon Butter Baked Tilapia — 122
Garlicky Shrimp Zucchini Pasta — 124
Pesto Shrimp Skewers with Cauliflower Mash — 125
Perfect Baked Cod — 126
Zucchini Ravioli — 129
Caprese Stuffed Avocados — 130

AMAZING SIDES — 132

Smashed Broccoli — 133
Twice-Baked Cauliflower — 134
Cheesy Baked Asparagus — 137
Mashed Cauliflower — 138
Bacon Ranch Sprouts — 140
Cheesy Brussels Sprouts Bake — 140
Magic Gnocchi — 141
Bacon Zucchini Fries — 141
Bacon Avocado Fries — 143
Loaded Cauliflower Salad — 144
Grilled Mushrooms — 147
Cauliflower Stuffing — 148

SUPER SNACKS — 150

- Cucumber Sushi — 151
- Zucchini Parmesan Chips — 151
- Greek Yogurt Onion Dip — 152
- Creamy Avocado Dip — 152
- Burger Fat Bombs — 153
- Mozzarella Sticks with Dill–Yogurt Dip — 154
- Avocado Chips — 157
- Loaded Cheese Nachos — 158
- Brussels Sprouts Chips — 161
- Bacon Asparagus Bites — 162
- Cauliflower Pizza Bites — 162
- Buffalo Chicken Celery Boats — 163
- Bell Pepper Nachos — 163

BREAD, BUNS & MORE — 164

- Low–Carb Sandwich Bread — 165
- Zucchini Taco Shells — 165
- Jalapeño Popper Bread — 166
- Burger Buns — 166
- Garlic Bread — 167
- Cloud Bread (Three Ways!) — 168
- Cheesy Cauli Bread — 170
- Broccoli Cheesy Bread — 171
- Cauliflower Garlic Bread — 172

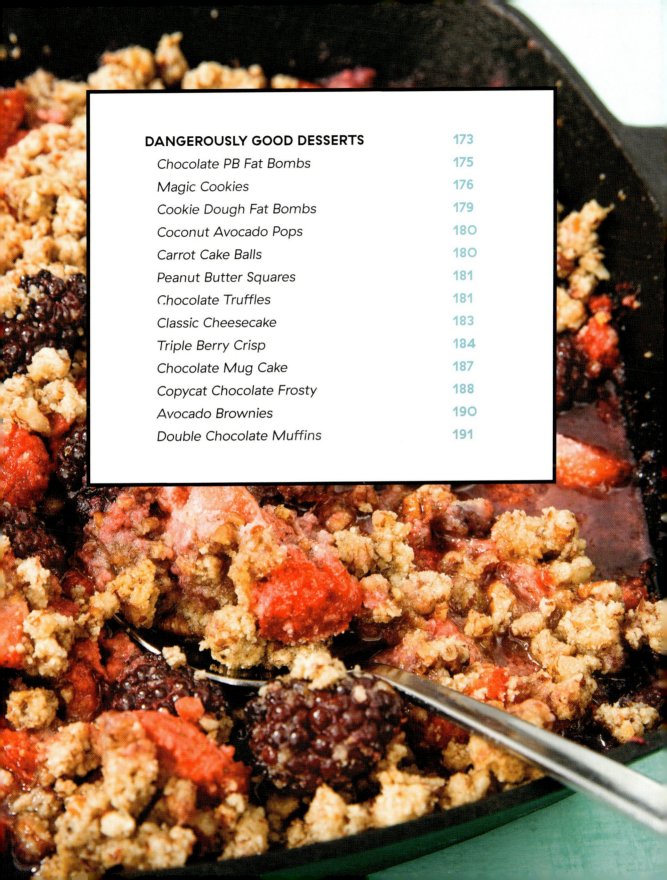

DANGEROUSLY GOOD DESSERTS 173
  Chocolate PB Fat Bombs 175
  Magic Cookies 176
  Cookie Dough Fat Bombs 179
  Coconut Avocado Pops 180
  Carrot Cake Balls 180
  Peanut Butter Squares 181
  Chocolate Truffles 181
  Classic Cheesecake 183
  Triple Berry Crisp 184
  Chocolate Mug Cake 187
  Copycat Chocolate Frosty 188
  Avocado Brownies 190
  Double Chocolate Muffins 191

EVERYTHING YOU NEED TO KNOW ABOUT KETO

THE SECRET TO SATISFYING YOUR CARB CRAVINGS

No doubt you have at least one friend who is doing the keto diet. Or maybe you've read about the long list of celebrities who swear by the eating approach: Halle Berry, Alicia Vikander, Mama June, Vinny Guadagnino, Kourtney Kardashian, Tim Tebow, Megan Fox, and Jenna Jameson.

Short for "ketogenic," the keto diet speeds weight loss with a macronutrient formula that dials down the carbs while dialing up the fat.

And the results are impressive, with people posting their body transformation photos all over Instagram, and continually boasting how they eat until they feel satisfied and get to eat damn yummy dishes that seem to always feature one food: bacon. Everyone loves bacon, after all. Except vegetarians. And, of course, swine.

But there's just one problem—and it's a biggie.

Carbs.

You no doubt picked up this guide because the moment you think about ditching carbs is the moment you feel driven to stuff a fresh piece of bread into your mouth.

Or pizza. Or a cookie. Or a slice of pizza followed by a chocolate-covered pretzel and a cookie...with some ice cream. Or about 150 other foods.

And there's nothing wrong with that.

Because the flavor and texture of high-carbohydrate foods makes life worth living.

HOW TO DITCH CARBS AND FEEL LIKE YOU'RE EATING THEM, TOO

The editors of *Delish* worked closely with the editors of *Women's Health* to find a way for you to achieve keto weight loss without giving up the carby textures and flavors you've come to adore.

In this guide, you'll learn dozens of cooking hacks from the *Delish* test kitchen (geniuses, they are). Plus, you'll get science-based advice from *Women's Health* as well as a 21-day menu, complete with meal prep tasks and a shopping list—created by keto coach and Registered Dietitian Nutritionist Lara Clevenger, M.S.H., R.D.N., C.P.T. Clevenger embraced the keto diet several years ago in an effort to combat her family history of metabolic syndrome, cancer, obesity, and high blood pressure. The diet helped her to drop pounds, sleep better, and gain energy, and it turned her into an evangelist. She now recommends the diet to her clients and co-runs The Keto Queens website.

When you combine Lara's guidance with *Women's Health's* expertise and *Delish's* recipes, you end up with everything you need to eat satisfying foods while still ditching the pounds.

On this plan you can and should eat pizza. And tacos. And lasagna. And pancakes. And even grilled cheese. And waffles. And fried chicken.

You'll just prepare them differently, using low-carb ingredients that have the taste and mouthfeel of the carbs you love—but without the actual carbs.

Get ready to dig in.

7 REASONS YOU'LL LOVE THE KETO DIET

Short for the "ketogenic diet," keto eating plans are high in fat (60 to 75 percent of your calories), moderate in protein (15 to 30 percent), and low in carbs (5 to 10 percent). This breakdown sends your body into a state called ketosis. That merely means that your body is breaking down fat into compounds called ketones that your cells can burn for energy. And burning fat for energy can lead to major results in the weight loss department.

Because of ketosis, you may be able to:

1. Double your weight loss.
People who followed the keto diet for two years lost more than twice as much weight (27 pounds vs. 10 pounds) than people on a standard low-calorie diet, according to a study of 45 obese people published in the journal *Endocrine*. The keto dieters also lost 4.5 inches from their waists, compared to the 1.6 inches of low-calorie dieters.

2. Lose fat, not muscle.
Keto helps you shrink abdominal fat while preserving the muscle mass you need to keep your metabolism humming, found a study published in the *Journal of Nutrition*.

3. Stop feeling so hungry all the time.
The keto diet increases satiety and curbs cravings. People usually reduce their daily caloric intake to about 1,500 calories a day (naturally) because the diet makes them feel fuller sooner—and for a longer period of time.

4. Kick start your metabolism.
It takes more energy to process and burn fat and protein than it does with carbs, so you will burn slightly more calories—even if you have not increased your exercise—while on the keto diet.

5. Reduce inflammation.
The keto diet drives down several biomarkers of inflammation, research shows. Because inflammation is predictive of other diseases, lower inflammation equals greater overall health.

6. Improve insulin sensitivity.
This is really a simple equation. When you eat fewer carbs, your blood glucose goes down, which in turn lowers your insulin levels. Lower insulin levels help to improve insulin sensitivity, finds research.

7. Lower cholesterol levels.
In one study, total cholesterol dropped throughout the 24 weeks study participants were following a keto diet. HDL (the good cholesterol) improved, while LDL (the bad kind) and triglycerides dropped.

YOUR KETO QUESTIONS, ANSWERED

You have questions? We have answers.

Who invented keto? Decades ago, doctors at the Mayo Clinic in Minnesota knew that low blood sugar—induced by fasting—could help control epilepsy, but they also knew straight fasting was not a therapy most patients could stick to. So they created a diet meant to trick your body into thinking it was starving (without the whole not having enough sustenance to live part). This high-fat, low-carbohydrate diet was called the ketogenic diet, after the "ketones" that seemed to have an anti-seizure effect.

Then, in the 1970s, Dr. Robert Atkins noticed that people who started following the keto diet also started losing weight. He started to prescribe keto to his overweight patients. But he didn't call it keto. He called it the Atkins diet. And it's still around.

Why is it called "keto"? The diet causes the body to release ketones into the bloodstream.

How does it help with weight loss? Our cells use blood sugar—which comes from dietary carbohydrates—to create energy. But when blood sugar levels remain low—as they do when you are consuming fewer than 50 daily grams of carbs—the body breaks down stored fat (yay!) into molecules called "ketones." Cells then burn these ketones for energy, and your weight goes down.

How much will I lose? Everyone is different, but keto followers claim they drop one to two pounds a week.

How long does it take to induce fat-burning? It takes two to four days of consuming 20–50 grams of carbs a day before the body shifts into ketosis and starts using fat as fuel.

Should anyone not follow the keto diet? Yes. It's a good idea to talk to your doctor before starting any new eating approach, including this one. Though the keto diet is generally safe for otherwise healthy people, it should not be followed long term by people who have certain health conditions, including diabetes, high blood pressure, or kidney, heart, or liver disease.

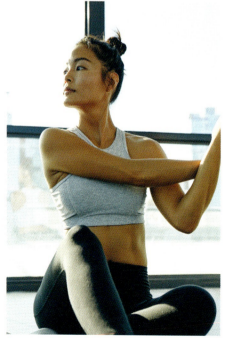

Are there side effects? Some people feel tired when their body initially hits ketosis. Other common issues: bad breath, nausea, vomiting, constipation, and sleep problems. (Most of these resolve after a few days.) *Women's Health* reported on keto breath, which is a funny phenomenon. When your body breaks down fat, it produces a lot of chemicals, including acetone, which stinks—literally. It makes your breath smell like nail polish remover. Thankfully, it's short lived. After two weeks, keto breath—along with other side effects—usually subsides.

How will it affect my workouts? Yes, you may feel more tired initially, but your energy will eventually rebound to better than when you started.

THE 3 RULES OF KETO FOR CARB LOVERS

In the 21-day plan, you'll find menus, shopping lists, and meal prep tips to help guide you. (Yup, we've done pretty much all the work for you!) But you'll probably also want to come up with your own keto meals. Follow this formula.

1. **Limit carbs to no more than 5 to 10 percent of your total calories.** For most people, that means eating no more than 50 grams of carbs a day (some strict keto dieters even opt for just 20 grams a day). Most of those should come from non-starchy, high-fiber veggies—think broccoli, asparagus, leafy greens, bell peppers, and cauliflower. Starchy vegetables you should definitely avoid: potatoes and other root vegetables, carrots, peas, and winter squash. Aim for 3 to 5 servings of non-starchy vegetables a day.

2. **Keep protein to about 15 to 30 percent of your daily calories.** For most people, that's somewhere between 75 to 150 grams and it's an easy number to reach. Just 3 ounces of salmon or tuna gets you to 21 grams. A ½ cup of cottage cheese nets you 14.

3. **Make sure 60 to 75 percent of your calories come from fat.** Yes, it sounds like a lot, but most of this fat should be the healthy kind, like omega-3 fatty acids in salmon and the monounsaturated fats in olive oil and avocados.

HOW TO ACE WEEK 1

Okay, so the keto diet is awesome, but we're not going to lie. The first few days are not necessarily great.

Your body needs to exhaust its stored glucose (glycogen) before it will shift into ketosis, a process that takes three to four days. This carb withdrawal can lead to a group of symptoms—feeling wiped out, as well as nausea, mental fog, headaches, diarrhea, and cramps—often referred to as "the keto flu."

Luckily, the keto flu doesn't usually last more than a week—which is coincidentally when you'll probably start to see the number on the scale go down.

To overcome these problems, use this advice:

Eat 3 to 5 servings of veggies a day. The fiber in the veggies will help to bulk up your stools, and help reduce bathroom trips. Just make sure you're eating non-starchy veggies such as broccoli and spinach rather than carb-rich starchy ones such as potatoes.

Stay hydrated. Drink half your body weight in ounces. So, if you weigh 150 pounds, you'll need 75 ounces, which is 9 to 10 cups of water a day.

Don't shy away from salt. (Unless, of course, you're under doctor's orders to do so.) Just before your body switches to burning fat for fuel, it will burn through all of your available stores of carbohydrate, including glycogen. This leads to your body releasing water and sodium, and the sodium deprivation can lead to light-headedness, dizziness, and fatigue with exercise. The keto diet can cause your body to lose its salt stores, so you'll need 3 to 5 grams of sodium a day, or about half a teaspoon to or 2 ½ teaspoons of salt. A couple daily cups of broth or bouillon will do the trick, and you only need to do this for the first few weeks of the keto diet.

Load up on minerals. This will help to combat muscle cramps and headaches, both of which are common during the early days of the keto diet, says Lara. Gravitate toward low-carb, mineral-rich foods, such as green leafy veggies, avocado, salmon, cabbage, zucchini, nuts, and seeds. You can also take 300–400 mg of magnesium glycinate at bedtime and 300–400 mg of potassium citrate daily. Speak with your doctor before taking any supplements.

Don't rely too much on medicine. While you may be tempted to reach for antidiarrheal medicine like Imodium, resist the urge. That won't treat the underlying problem. Instead, it's smarter to stick with the other advice in this chapter.

Cut back on the artificial sweeteners. If you're tempted to replace sugar with non-nutritive sweeteners (think: aspartame or Splenda) and sugar alcohols (like sorbitol or xylitol), think again. Both can lead to digestive troubles.

Consume fermented foods. Keto causes you to cut out important sources of fiber, like whole grains and fruits, which can make you feel pretty backed up.

That's where fermented veggies come in: They act as a probiotic to support healthy bacteria in your gut, which helps to keep you regular. Try adding more to your diet through kimchi, sauerkraut, or pickles. Kefir and yogurt are great probiotic options, too.

7 KETO-APPROVED FOODS AND SNACKS FOR CARB LOVERS

You'll be happy that these foods are not off limits on keto. Yum.

1. **Blackberries:** Blackberries have an impressive amount of fiber—nearly 2 grams per ¼ cup. That serving size also has 1.5 grams of net carbs, so you can definitely add these to your morning yogurt.
2. **Raspberries:** Per ¼ cup, you'll get about 1.5 grams of net carbs, per the USDA. Toss them in a smoothie, or, even better: whip up heavy whipping cream and toss a few berries on top for a keto-friendly dessert.
3. **Strawberries:** A ¼ cup of strawberry halves contains a little more than 2 grams of net carbs—or about 10 percent of your daily limit if you're aiming for 20 grams of net carbs a day.
4. **Avocado:** Yep, this creamy delight is actually a fruit—and it's a keto diet Godsend. Not only does a half of an avocado contain a glorious 15 grams of heart-healthy fat, but it has less than 2 grams of net carbs.
5. **Keto Frappuccino:** Order a Frapp made with unsweetened almond, coconut milk, or heavy cream, and whatever sugar-free flavoring is your pleasure (vanilla, caramel, hazelnut — you get the idea).
6. **Keto Fat Bombs:** Check out the recipes starting on page 175. As the name implies, these glorious little snacks are high in fat and low in carbs, so you can be on point with your diet, even when you indulge.
7. **Keto Pasta:** Explore Skinny Shirataki Noodles to get the pasta experience without the carbs.

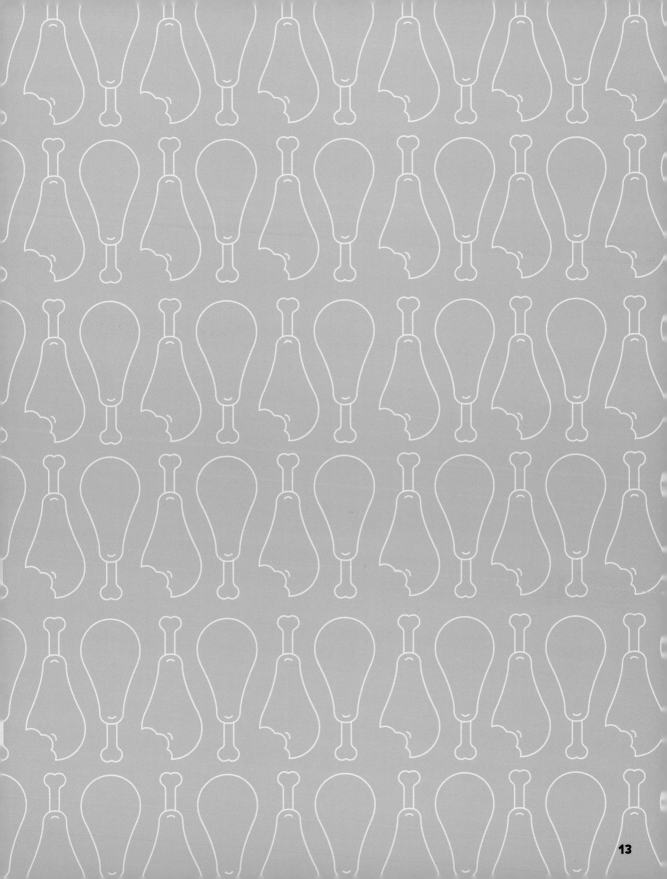

HOW TO FOLLOW THE 21-DAY PLAN

Jumping on the keto bandwagon can be overwhelming at first, and we TOTALLY get that. So that's why we worked with keto queen Lara to create this super easy 21-day plan. With her meal plans, grocery lists, and meal prep tasks, following the keto diet has never been easier!

Meal Plans. Each day you'll eat about 1,750–1,850 calories, and 20–30 grams net carbs. Lara made these plans super simple to minimize your kitchen time.

Grocery Lists. Just follow the list and you're good to go. Don't get intimidated by the length of the first grocery list. You're going to need to stock up on the keto pantry essentials like Swerve sweeteners, Rao's marinara, bacon, almond flour, and more. Once you have all your go-to pantry items, your lists get smaller, so you can get in and out of the grocery store in no time.

Meal Prep Tasks. When you meal prep, the rest of your week instantly becomes so much easier. Lara's meal prep tips are genius, too, and they can save you an hour or more of kitchen time during your work week!

WHAT HAPPENS AFTER 21 DAYS

We're still here for you once you've finished the 21-day plan.

Starting on page 32, you'll find 100+ recipes that tame your carb cravings. Dig into delicious recipes like Loaded Cheese Nachos (page 158), Crispy Chicken and Waffles (page 97), Cheesy Lasagna (page 75), and Triple Berry Crisp (page 184). We've included the nutritional information for each recipe to make it easy for you to plan your meals. To figure out the net carbs of a recipe, subtract the fiber from the total carbohydrates. Most of these recipes have no more than 10 grams net carbs per serving, while some have almost none at all! We provided so many tasty options so that you'll never feel bored or limited. Pick what works best for you.

WEEK 1

GROCERY LIST

If your budget allows, aim to buy grass-fed beef and dairy products.

MEAT & PROTEIN
- ☐ 2 pounds cubed top round beef roast
- ☐ 5 ounces ribeye
- ☐ 1 rotisserie chicken
- ☐ 1 (3-ounce) chicken thigh with skin
- ☐ 2½ pounds boneless, skinless chicken breasts
- ☐ 2 ounces uncured turkey breast
- ☐ 2 pounds ground turkey
- ☐ 2 ounces uncured ham
- ☐ 2 pounds uncured bacon
- ☐ 3 dozen large eggs

DAIRY
- ☐ 1 pint whole milk
- ☐ 1 pint heavy cream
- ☐ 1 (4-ounce) container blue cheese or goat cheese
- ☐ 1 (1-pound) box butter
- ☐ 2 (8-ounce) bags shredded cheddar
- ☐ 1 (8-ounce) bag shredded Monterey Jack
- ☐ 2 (8-ounce) bags shredded mozzarella
- ☐ 2 (8-ounce) containers grated Parmesan
- ☐ 1 (16-ounce) container sour cream
- ☐ 1 (16-ounce) container ricotta
- ☐ 1 (10-ounce) bag mozzarella string cheese
- ☐ 1 (6-ounce) container full-fat Greek yogurt
- ☐ 1 (8-ounce) package cream cheese

PRODUCE
- ☐ 1 head Boston or Bibb lettuce
- ☐ 1 head romaine lettuce
- ☐ 1 (10-ounce) package spinach
- ☐ 1 (16-ounce) bunch asparagus
- ☐ 1 lemon
- ☐ 1 lime
- ☐ 1 jalapeño
- ☐ 1 cucumber
- ☐ 4 medium zucchinis
- ☐ 2 scallions
- ☐ 1 red bell pepper
- ☐ 2 yellow onions
- ☐ 1 head garlic
- ☐ 4 avocados
- ☐ 2 medium tomatoes

continued

WEEK 1

GROCERY LIST, CONT.

- ☐ 2 large heads cauliflower
- ☐ 1 (12-ounce) package riced cauliflower
- ☐ 1 (16-ounce) package sliced mushrooms
- ☐ 2 (.75-ounce) packages fresh chives
- ☐ 1 (.75-ounce) package fresh dill
- ☐ 1 small bunch cilantro
- ☐ 1 small bunch parsley
- ☐ 1 (6-ounce) package raspberries
- ☐ 2 (6-ounce) packages blackberries
- ☐ 1 pint strawberries

PANTRY

- ☐ 1 (750-milliliter) bottle avocado oil
- ☐ 1 (750-milliliter) bottle olive oil
- ☐ 1 (48-ounce) bottle canola oil
- ☐ 1 (16-ounce) bottle MCT oil (or coconut oil)
- ☐ 1 (12-ounce) jar avocado oil mayonnaise
- ☐ 1 (16-ounce) bottle ranch dressing (avocado oil based, if available)
- ☐ 1 (6-ounce) can tomato paste
- ☐ 1 (28-ounce) can crushed tomatoes
- ☐ 1 (16-ounce) bottle white vinegar
- ☐ 1 (7-ounce) can chipotle chiles in adobo
- ☐ 1 (2.25-ounce) can sliced black olives
- ☐ 1 (10-ounce) jar green olives
- ☐ 1 (36-ounce) jar dill pickle spears
- ☐ 1 (10-ounce) bag pecans
- ☐ 1 (9-ounce) bag macadamia nuts
- ☐ 1 (5.25-ounce) bag sunflower seeds
- ☐ 1 (4-ounce) bag pork rinds
- ☐ 1 (32-ounce) container beef broth
- ☐ 1 (5-ounce) bottle soy sauce
- ☐ 1 bottle chili powder
- ☐ 1 bottle cumin
- ☐ 1 bottle garlic powder
- ☐ 1 (4-ounce) bottle stevia extract
- ☐ 1 bottle cinnamon
- ☐ 1 bottle red pepper flakes
- ☐ 1 bottle sweet or smoked paprika
- ☐ 1 bottle Italian seasoning
- ☐ 1 (11-ounce) can ground coffee
- ☐ 1 (100-gram) bar of 90% dark chocolate or stevia-sweetened chocolate
- ☐ 1 (12-ounce) bag Swerve confectioners' sugar
- ☐ 1 (4-ounce) bottle vanilla extract
- ☐ 1 (48-ounce) bag almond flour
- ☐ 1 (14-ounce) bag ground flax seed
- ☐ 1 (9-ounce) bag Lily's or stevia-sweetened chocolate chips
- ☐ 1 (8-ounce) container baking powder

MEAL PREP TASKS

Store all your prepped items in air-tight containers. Store perishable items in your refrigerator.

- Chop and store 2 cups romaine lettuce
- Store in individual bags or containers:
  - 1 ounce cheddar
  - 2 ounces cucumber, sliced
  - 2 ounces sliced turkey breast
  - 2 tablespoons sunflower seeds
  - 2 tablespoons ranch dressing
  - 1 tablespoon chopped white onion
  - 10 macadamia nuts
  - 10 green olives
  - 1.5 ounces pecans
- Make buns for Spicy Chicken Sandwich (page 54)
- Make Cookie Dough Fat Bombs (page 179), make on day 5

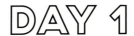

DAY 1

BREAKFAST

Bacon and Eggs with Avocado

In a large skillet over medium-high heat, cook 1 ounce of uncured bacon until crisp. Remove from skillet and drain on paper towel-lined plate. In the same skillet over medium-high heat, heat 1 teaspoon of avocado oil. In a small bowl, whisk together 3 large eggs. Add eggs to skillet and cook until set, about 3 to 5 minutes. Serve with 2 ounces of sliced avocado.

LUNCH

Turkey Club Salad

In a large bowl, combine 2 cups of romaine lettuce, chopped, 1 ounce of cheddar cheese, 2 ounces of turkey breast, 2 ounces of cucumber, 2 ounces of avocado, sliced, 2 tablespoons of sunflower seeds, and 2 tablespoons of ranch dressing.

DINNER

Crispy Chicken and Waffles (page 97)

DESSERT

Triple Berry Crisp (page 184)

DAY 2

BREAKFAST

Spinach and Cheese Omelet

In a large skillet over medium heat, heat 1 tablespoon of avocado oil. In a small bowl, whisk together 2 large eggs. Add the eggs, ½ ounce of cheddar, 2 cups of spinach, and 1 tablespoon of chopped onion to the skillet. Cook until eggs are set, about 3 to 5 minutes.

LUNCH

Leftover Crispy Chicken and Waffles

Serve with 3 dill pickle spears and 10 macadamia nuts.

DINNER

Slow-Cooked Beef Stroganoff (page 76)

SNACK

10 green olives

1.5 ounces pecans

DAY 3

BREAKFAST

Perfect Pancakes (page 37)

3 pancakes topped with 2 tablespoons of butter

10 blackberries

LUNCH

Leftover Slow-Cooked Beef Stroganoff

SNACK

Mozzarella Sticks with Dill-Yogurt Dip (page 154)

DINNER

Pan-Seared Ribeye with Asparagus

Heat grill or grill pan to high. Season both sides of a 5-ounce ribeye with kosher salt and pepper. Grill 4 to 6 minutes on each side. Meanwhile, in a small skillet, heat 1 tablespoon of butter. Cook 8 medium trimmed asparagus spears until tender, about 5 minutes.

DAY 4

BREAKFAST

Bulletproof Coffee + Cauli Breakfast Hash (page 50)

8 ounces brewed coffee blended with 1 tablespoon of MCT oil (or coconut oil) and 2 tablespoons heavy cream.

LUNCH

Leftover Mozzarella Sticks with Herb Yogurt + Chicken Thigh

In a small skillet over medium heat, heat 1 teaspoon of avocado oil. Add 1 (3-ounce) chicken thigh to the pan skin-side down. Cook until golden and seared, about 5 minutes, then flip. Cook until temperature reaches 165°, about 10 minutes. Serve with 1 ounce of cheddar.

DINNER

Cheesy Lasagna (page 75) **+ Bacon Zucchini Fries** (page 141)

Serve fries with 2 tablespoons ranch dressing.

DESSERT

Triple Berry Crisp (page 184)

DAY 5

BREAKFAST

Leftover Perfect Pancakes

3 pancakes topped with 1 tablespoon butter

10 blackberries

LUNCH

Leftover Cheesy Lasagna + Bacon Zucchini Fries (2 servings)

DINNER

Spicy Chicken Sandwich

(page 54)

DESSERT

½ Ounce 90% Dark Chocolate or Stevia-Sweetened Chocolate

DAY 6

BREAKFAST

Bulletproof Coffee + Cauli Breakfast Hash (page 50)

8 ounces brewed coffee blended with 1 tablespoon of MCT oil (or coconut oil) and 2 tablespoons heavy cream.

LUNCH

Leftover Spicy Chicken Sandwich

DINNER

Loaded Cheese Nachos

(page 158)

Serve with leftover Bacon Zucchini Fries (2 servings).

DAY 7

BREAKFAST

Bulletproof Coffee + Taco Brunch Casserole

(page 41)

8 ounces brewed coffee blended with 1 tablespoon of MCT oil (or coconut oil) and 2 tablespoons heavy cream.

LUNCH

Leftover Loaded Cheese Nachos (1 serving)

Serve with 2 ounces uncured ham.

DINNER

Chicken Lettuce Cups

Add 3 ounces of rotisserie chicken, 3 large leaves of Boston or Bibb lettuce, 2 ounces of avocado and 1 ounce of crumbled blue cheese or goat cheese. Drizzle with 2 tablespoons ranch/blue cheese dressing.

DESSERT

3 Cookie Dough Fat Bombs

(page 179)

WEEK 2

GROCERY LIST

If your budget allows it, aim to buy grass-fed beef and dairy products.

MEAT & PROTEIN
- ☐ 1 pound skirt steak
- ☐ ½ pound sirloin steak
- ☐ 1 pound 80/20 ground beef
- ☐ 1 rotisserie chicken
- ☐ 2 (8-ounce) packages uncured ham
- ☐ 3 pounds uncured bacon
- ☐ 1 (12-ounce) package sausage
- ☐ 1 pound salmon fillets
- ☐ 1 pound medium or large shrimp, peeled and deveined
- ☐ 3 dozen large eggs

PRODUCE
- ☐ 1 head of Bibb or Boston lettuce
- ☐ 1 (10-ounce) package spinach
- ☐ ½ pound Brussels sprouts
- ☐ 2 large heads cauliflower
- ☐ 1 head broccoli
- ☐ 7 medium zucchinis
- ☐ 1 (8-ounce) bunch asparagus spears
- ☐ 3 large bell peppers
- ☐ 3 medium onions
- ☐ 1 shallot
- ☐ 4 avocados
- ☐ 2 lemons
- ☐ 1 pint cherry tomatoes
- ☐ 1 bunch fresh parsley
- ☐ 1 (.75-ounce) package fresh thyme leaves
- ☐ 1 (.75-ounce) package fresh rosemary
- ☐ 1 (.75-ounce) package fresh chives

DAIRY
- ☐ 1 (1-pound) box butter
- ☐ 1 (8-ounce) bag shredded cheddar
- ☐ 1 (8-ounce) bag shredded Monterey Jack
- ☐ 8 ounces provolone
- ☐ 1 (8-ounce) block cheddar
- ☐ 1 (16-ounce) container sour cream
- ☐ 2 pints heavy cream

PANTRY
- ☐ 1 (24-ounce) jar tomato sauce, such as Rao's Homemade Pasta Sauce
- ☐ 1 (4-ounce) container grated Parmesan cheese
- ☐ 1 (6-ounce) package pepperoni
- ☐ 1 (5-ounce) container hot sauce
- ☐ 1 (12-ounce) bottle Dijon mustard
- ☐ 1 (12-ounce) bottle Caesar dressing (avocado oil based, if possible)
- ☐ 1 (8-ounce) container cocoa powder
- ☐ 1 (16-ounce) jar unsweetened peanut butter, such as Smucker's Creamy Natural Peanut Butter
- ☐ 1 (8-ounce) container baking soda
- ☐ 1 bottle dried oregano

WEEK 2

MEAL PREP TASKS

Store all your prepped items in air-tight containers. Store perishable items in your refrigerator.

- Make Burger Buns (page 166)
- Make Ham, Egg & Cheese Roll-Ups (page 45)
- Trim asparagus spears
- Slice peppers and onion for No-Carb Philly Cheesesteak (page 72)
- Make Copycat Chocolate Frosty (page 188), store in freezer and thaw in fridge when needed
- Measure out ½ ounce of pecans and 1 ounce of pecans
- Chop 3 cups of broccoli
- Make Avocado Brownies (page 190)
- Slice Brussels sprouts for the Brussels Sprouts Chips (page 161)

DAY 8

BREAKFAST

Leftover Taco Brunch Casserole

LUNCH

Rotisserie Chicken Sandwich

Halve 1 Burger Bun (page 166) and spread 1 tablespoon of mayonnaise on each side. Top with 3 ounces of leftover rotisserie chicken, 3 dill pickle spears, and 1 to 2 large pieces of lettuce.

DINNER

Pizza-Stuffed Zucchini

(page 83)

DESSERT

1 Cookie Dough Fat Bomb

(page 179)

DAY 9

BREAKFAST

2 Ham, Egg & Cheese Roll-Ups (page 45)

LUNCH

Leftover Pizza-Stuffed Zucchini (1 serving)

DINNER

Keto Cheeseburger

Preheat a grill or grill pan to medium-high heat. Grill 1 (3-ounce) beef patty until cooked to your liking, about 4 minutes per side. Halve 1 Burger Bun (page 166). Top with burger, 1 ounce of cheddar, 2 large lettuce leaves, and 3 dill pickle spears.

DAY 10

BREAKFAST

Bacon Weave Breakfast Tacos (page 48)

LUNCH

Lettuce Burger + Twice-Baked Cauliflower

(page 134)

Preheat a grill or grill pan to medium-high heat. Grill 1 (3-ounce) beef patty until cooked to your liking, about 4 minutes per side. Top 1 large lettuce leaf with burger, 1 ounce of cheddar, and 2 ounces of sliced avocado.

DINNER

Rosemary-Dijon Salmon

(page 112)

Cook asparagus spears in 1 teaspoon of avocado oil.

DESSERT

Chocolate Mug Cake (page 187)

DAY 11

BREAKFAST

Bulletproof Coffee + 2 Leftover Ham, Egg & Cheese Roll-Ups

8 ounces brewed coffee blended with 1 tablespoon of MCT oil (or coconut oil) and 2 tablespoons heavy cream.

LUNCH

Leftover Twice-Baked Cauliflower and Rosemary-Dijon Salmon

DINNER

No-Carb Philly Cheesesteak

(page 72)

DESSERT

Copycat Chocolate Frosty

(page 188)

½ ounce pecans

DAY 12

BREAKFAST

Bulletproof Coffee + Leftover Bacon Weave Breakfast Taco

8 ounces brewed coffee blended with 1 tablespoon of MCT oil (or coconut oil) and 2 tablespoons heavy cream.

LUNCH

Leftover No-Carb Philly Cheesesteak

DINNER

Rotisserie Chicken + Broccoli and Cheese

In a large skillet over medium heat, heat 1 tablespoon of avocado oil. Add 2 cups of chopped broccoli. Cook until tender, about 5 minutes. Push broccoli to one side of the pan and add 3 ounces of leftover rotisserie chicken. Top both chicken and broccoli with 1 ounce of cheddar. Cover and cook until cheddar is melted, about 1 minute.

DESSERT

Leftover Copycat Chocolate Frosty

DAY 13

BREAKFAST

Bulletproof Coffee + Eggs & Sausage Scramble

8 ounces brewed coffee blended with 1 tablespoon of MCT oil (or coconut oil) and 2 tablespoons heavy cream.

In a medium skillet over medium heat, melt 1 tablespoon of butter. In a small bowl, whisk 2 large eggs. Add 2 ounces of cooked breakfast sausage to the skillet. Add eggs and cook until set, about 3 minutes, stirring occasionally.

LUNCH

4 Ounces Leftover Rotisserie Chicken With Brussels Sprouts Chips (page 161)

1 tablespoon Caesar or ranch dressing to dip chips

DINNER

Garlicky Shrimp Zucchini Pasta (page 124)

DESSERT

Avocado Brownies (page 190)

DAY 14

BREAKFAST

Bulletproof Coffee + Cauli Breakfast Hash (page 50)

8 ounces brewed coffee blended with 1 tablespoon of MCT oil (or coconut oil) and 2 tablespoons heavy cream.

LUNCH

Leftover Garlicky Shrimp Zucchini Pasta

SNACK

1 ounce pecans

DINNER

Sirloin Steak with Leftover Brussels Sprouts Chips

Preheat a grill or grill pan to high heat. Season 6 ounces of sirloin steak with salt and pepper on both sides. Grill 4 to 6 minutes on both sides. Save 2 ounces of steak for breakfast tomorrow. Serve Brussels Sprouts Chips with 1 tablespoon of Caesar or ranch dressing.

DESSERT

Leftover Avocado Brownie

WEEK 3

GROCERY LIST

If your budget allows it, aim to buy grass-fed beef and dairy products.

MEAT & PROTEIN
- ☐ 1 pound 80/20 ground beef
- ☐ 8 all-beef uncured hot dogs
- ☐ 1 rotisserie chicken
- ☐ 1 pound pork loin chops
- ☐ 3 pounds uncured bacon
- ☐ 2 (8-ounce) packages uncured ham
- ☐ 4 ounces uncured salami or pepperoni
- ☐ 1 pound mahi-mahi fillets
- ☐ 24 ounces skin-on salmon fillets
- ☐ 12 ounces lump crab meat
- ☐ 2 dozen large eggs

DAIRY
- ☐ 2 (1-pound) boxes butter
- ☐ 1 pint 100% grass-fed whole milk yogurt
- ☐ 1 (4-ounce) container goat cheese or blue cheese
- ☐ 2 (8-ounce) bags shredded cheddar
- ☐ 1 (8-ounce) bag shredded Monterey Jack
- ☐ 1 (8-ounce) bag shredded mozzarella
- ☐ 1 (8-ounce) package cream cheese
- ☐ 1 (6-ounce) container full-fat Greek yogurt

PRODUCE
- ☐ 1 head Butterhead lettuce
- ☐ 1 head broccoli
- ☐ 2 large heads cauliflower
- ☐ ½ pound Brussels sprouts
- ☐ ½ pound green beans
- ☐ 2 pounds asparagus
- ☐ 1 (8-ounce) package sliced mushrooms
- ☐ 3 avocados
- ☐ 2 tomatoes
- ☐ 1 medium zucchini
- ☐ 1 cucumber
- ☐ 2 small yellow onions
- ☐ 1 red onion
- ☐ 1 head garlic
- ☐ 1 red bell pepper
- ☐ 5 lemons
- ☐ 3 pints blackberries
- ☐ 1 pint strawberries
- ☐ 1 bunch fresh cilantro
- ☐ 1 small bunch fresh parsley
- ☐ 1 (.75-ounce) package fresh rosemary
- ☐ 2 (.75-ounce) packages fresh chives
- ☐ 1 (.75-ounce) package fresh dill

PANTRY
- ☐ 1 (6-ounce) bag walnut halves
- ☐ 2 ounces 90% dark chocolate or stevia-sweetened chocolate
- ☐ 1 (14-ounce) bottle yellow mustard
- ☐ 1 (10-ounce) can red enchilada sauce
- ☐ 1 bottle cayenne pepper

MEAL PREP TASKS

Store all your prepped items in airtight containers. Store perishable items in your refrigerator.

- 3 tablespoons chopped onion
- Trim and store 6 asparagus spears
- Make Double Chocolate Muffins (page 191)
- Store in individual bags or containers:
  - 3 ounces mushrooms, sliced
  - 1 (15-piece) portion and 1 (5-piece) portion walnut halves
  - 10 green olives
  - 2 (1-ounce) pieces dark chocolate
  - 2 bags of 10 blackberries and 1 bag of 15 blackberries
  - 10 macadamia nuts
  - 2 (2-ounce) servings of sliced strawberries, and 1 (3-ounce) serving of strawberries
  - 2 hard-boiled eggs
  - 1 ounce pecans

DAY 15

BREAKFAST

Steak and Egg Scramble

In a large skillet over medium heat, heat 2 teaspoons of avocado oil. Add 2 ounces of leftover sirloin steak, 2 tablespoons of chopped onions, and 3 ounces of sliced mushrooms to the skillet. Cook until onions and mushrooms have softened, about 5 minutes. In a small bowl whisk 2 large eggs. Add the eggs to skillet and cook until set, about 3 minutes, stirring occasionally.

LUNCH

2 Ta-Ketos (page 61) with 2 Ounces Avocado

Serve with 1 tablespoon of sour cream.

DINNER

Garlic Rosemary Pork Chops (page 88) + Asparagus

In a medium skillet over medium heat, melt 1 tablespoon of butter. Add 6 asparagus spears and cook until tender, about 5 minutes.

DESSERT

Leftover Avocado Brownie

DAY 16

BREAKFAST

Leftover Cauli Breakfast Hash

LUNCH

Charcuterie Plate

2.5 dill pickle spears

1 ounce cheddar cheese

15 walnut halves

2 ounces uncured ham

2 ounces avocado

10 green olives

DINNER

Leftover Garlic Rosemary Pork Chops + Twice Baked Cauliflower (page 134)

DESSERT

Dark Chocolate with Berries

1 ounce 90% dark chocolate or stevia-sweetened chocolate

10 blackberries

DAY 17

BREAKFAST

Bulletproof Coffee + Ham & Cheese Egg Cups (page 42)

8 ounces brewed coffee blended with 1 tablespoon of MCT oil (or coconut oil) and 2 tablespoons heavy cream

3 Ham & Cheese Egg Cups

LUNCH

Charcuterie Plate

2 ounces uncured salami or pepperoni

1 ounce crumbled goat cheese or blue cheese

15 blackberries

2.5 dill pickle spears

DINNER

Garlicky Lemon Mahi-Mahi (page 121) with Leftover Twice-Baked Cauliflower and Brussels Sprouts

In a medium skillet over medium-high heat, cook 4 ounces of Brussels sprouts in ½ tablespoon of avocado oil until tender, about 10 minutes.

DESSERT

Chocolate + Nuts

1 ounce 90% dark chocolate

10 macadamia nuts

DAY 18

BREAKFAST

Yogurt + Meat Roll Ups

In a small bowl combine ½ cup of yogurt with 2 ounces of sliced strawberries and stevia drops (if needed for sweetness).

Top 2 ounces of uncured salami or pepperoni with 1 ounce of goat cheese or blue cheese.

LUNCH

Leftover Garlicky Lemon Mahi-Mahi + Broccoli & Cheese

In a small skillet over medium heat, heat 1 teaspoon of avocado oil. Add ½ cup of chopped broccoli and ½ ounce of cheddar. Cook until broccoli is tender and cheese is melted, about 5 minutes.

DINNER

Low-Carb Garlic Bread Dogs

(page 62) **with Zucchini**

In a small skillet over medium heat, heat 1 teaspoon of avocado oil. Cook 1 sliced zucchini until tender, about 5 minutes. Serve hot dog with 1 tablespoon of mustard.

DESSERT

Double Chocolate Muffins

(page 191)

DAY 19

BREAKFAST

3 Leftover Ham & Cheese Egg Cups

Serve with 3 ounces strawberries

LUNCH

Leftover Low-Carb Garlic Bread Dogs

Combine ½ of a medium sliced cucumber with 1 tablespoon ranch dressing. Serve Keto Dog with 1 tablespoon mustard.

DINNER

Grilled Salmon + Lemony Asparagus Foil Packs

(page 116)

DESSERT

Leftover Double Chocolate Muffins

DAY 20

BREAKFAST

Leftover Double Chocolate Muffin + Strawberries & Yogurt

In a small bowl, combine 2 ounces of strawberries with ½ cup of yogurt and stevia drops (if needed for sweetness).

LUNCH

Leftover Grilled Salmon + Lemony Asparagus Foil Packs

Serve with 5 walnut halves.

DINNER

BLT Burgers (page 66)

Serve with 3 dill pickle spears.

DAY 21

BREAKFAST

Hard-Boiled Eggs + Nuts & Berries

2 hard-boiled eggs

10 blackberries

1 ounce pecans

LUNCH

Leftover BLT Burger

Serve with 3 dill pickle spears.

DINNER

Avocado Crab Boats (page 110) **with Buttery Green Beans**

In a small skillet over medium heat, melt 1 tablespoon of butter. Add 1 cup of green beans and cook until tender, about 5 minutes.

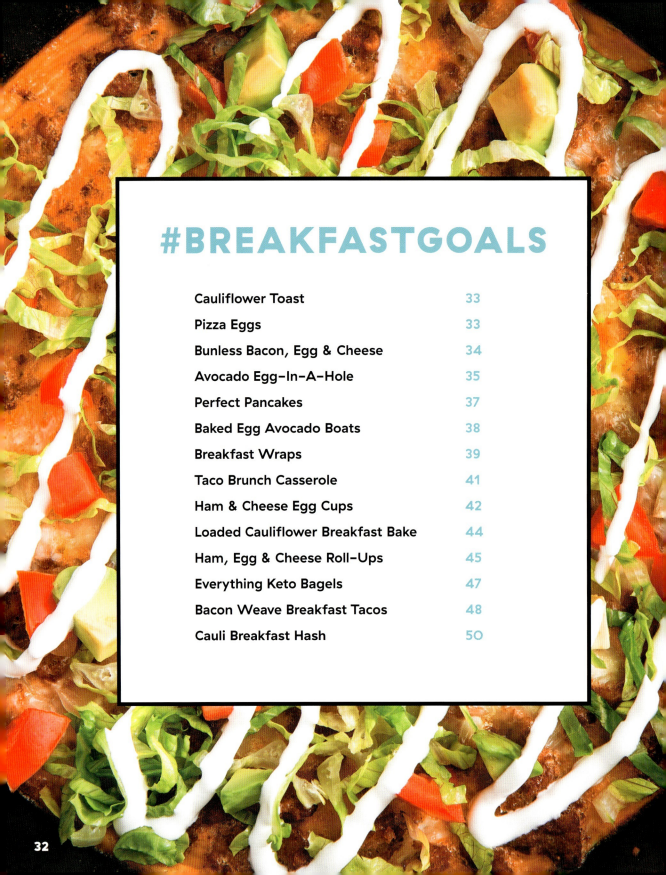

#BREAKFASTGOALS

Cauliflower Toast	33
Pizza Eggs	33
Bunless Bacon, Egg & Cheese	34
Avocado Egg-In-A-Hole	35
Perfect Pancakes	37
Baked Egg Avocado Boats	38
Breakfast Wraps	39
Taco Brunch Casserole	41
Ham & Cheese Egg Cups	42
Loaded Cauliflower Breakfast Bake	44
Ham, Egg & Cheese Roll-Ups	45
Everything Keto Bagels	47
Bacon Weave Breakfast Tacos	48
Cauli Breakfast Hash	50

CAULIFLOWER TOAST

TOTAL TIME: 45 MIN / SERVES 4 TO 6

This cauli toast is the best thing since, well, sliced bread.

1 medium head cauliflower

1 large egg

½ cup shredded cheddar

1 teaspoon garlic powder

Kosher salt

Freshly ground black pepper

1. Preheat oven to 425° and line a baking sheet with parchment paper. Finely grate cauliflower and transfer to a large bowl. Microwave on high, 8 minutes. Drain thoroughly with paper towels or a cheesecloth until mixture is dry.

2. Add egg, cheddar, and garlic powder to cauliflower bowl and season with salt and pepper. Mix until combined.

3. Form cauliflower into toast shapes on prepared baking sheet and bake until golden, 18 to 20 minutes.

4. Transfer to a plate and top with desired toppings, like mashed avocado, a fried egg, or bacon, lettuce and tomato.

Nutrition (per serving): 80 calories, 5 g protein, 5 g carbohydrates, 2 g fiber, 2 g sugars, 4 g fat, 2.5 g saturated fat, 100 mg sodium

PIZZA EGGS

TOTAL TIME: 10 MIN / SERVES 2

Pizza for breakfast?! Yes, please. This hack for mason jar lids helps transform your eggs into perfectly round "pizzas."

Cooking spray, for pan

2 large eggs

¼ cup pizza sauce, divided

¼ cup shredded mozzarella, divided

10 mini pepperoni

Freshly grated Parmesan, for garnish

Dried oregano, for garnish

Kosher salt

Freshly ground black pepper

1. Spray a medium skillet over medium heat with cooking spray, then spray the inside of a mason jar lid. Place mason jar lid in the center of skillet and crack an egg inside.

2. Top with half the pizza sauce, half the cheese, and half the pepperoni. Cover with lid and cook until egg white is set and cheese is melty, 4 to 5 minutes. Repeat with remaining ingredients. Top with Parmesan and oregano, season with salt and pepper, and serve.

Nutrition (per serving): 260 calories, 13 g protein, 4 g carbohydrates, 1 g fiber, 2 g sugar, 22 g fat, 7 g saturated fat, 550 mg sodium

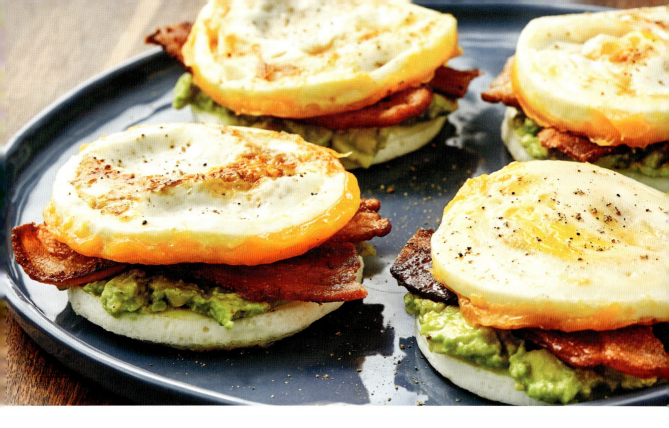

BUNLESS BACON, EGG & CHEESE

TOTAL TIME: 10 MIN / SERVES 1

The eggs become the bun in this genius low-carb twist on the classic breakfast sandwich.

2 large eggs
2 tablespoons water
¼ cup shredded cheddar
½ avocado, lightly mashed
2 slices cooked bacon

1. In a medium nonstick pan, place two mason jar lids (centers removed). Spray the entire pan with cooking spray and heat over medium heat. Crack eggs into the centers of the lids and lightly whisk with a fork to break up yolk.

2. Pour water around the lids and cover the pan. Cook, letting the eggs steam, until the whites are cooked through, about 3 minutes. Remove lid and top one egg with cheddar. Cook until the cheese is slightly melted, about 1 minute more.

3. Invert the egg bun without the cheese onto the plate. Top with mashed avocado and cooked bacon. Top with the cheesy egg bun, cheese-side down. Eat with fork and knife.

Nutrition (per serving): 460 calories, 27 g protein, 7 g carbohydrates, 5 g fiber, 1 g sugar, 36 g fat, 13 g saturated fat, 600 mg sodium

AVOCADO EGG-IN-A-HOLE

TOTAL TIME: 20 MIN / SERVES 4

Just because you're ditching bread doesn't mean you don't get to enjoy this childhood favorite. Avocado slices become the perfect nest for a fried egg. After hollowing out the avo, dice up the scraps and use them as a garnish.

2 avocados
2 tablespoons butter, divided
4 large eggs
Kosher salt
Freshly ground black pepper
¼ cup shredded cheddar
2 slices cooked bacon, crumbled
2 green onions, sliced

1. Cut each avocado in half and remove pit. Lay avocado halves on their sides and carefully cut lengthwise into 2 thick slices each. Hollow out middles with a paring knife.

2. In a large, nonstick skillet over medium-low heat, melt 1 tablespoon butter. Place the eight avocado slices into skillet and crack an egg into the center of each. Season with salt and pepper.

3. Cover skillet and cook until egg is cooked to your desired doneness, about 5 minutes for a just runny egg. Sprinkle cheese on top of each slice, cover with lid again and cook until the cheese is melted, 1 minute more.

4. Repeat with remaining ingredients. Garnish with bacon and green onions.

Nutrition (per serving): 340 calories, 12 g protein, 10 g carbohydrates, 7 g fiber, 1 g sugar, 30 g fat, 9 g saturated fat, 240 mg sodium

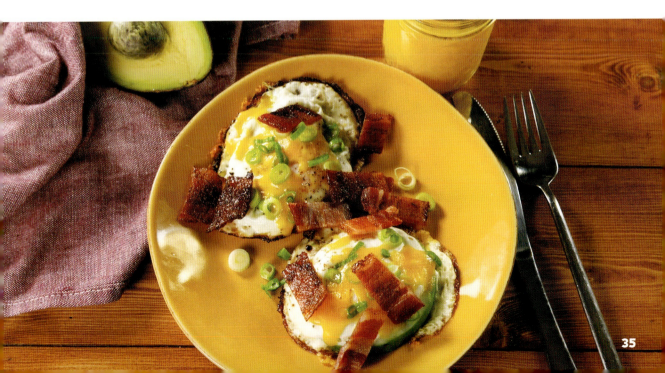

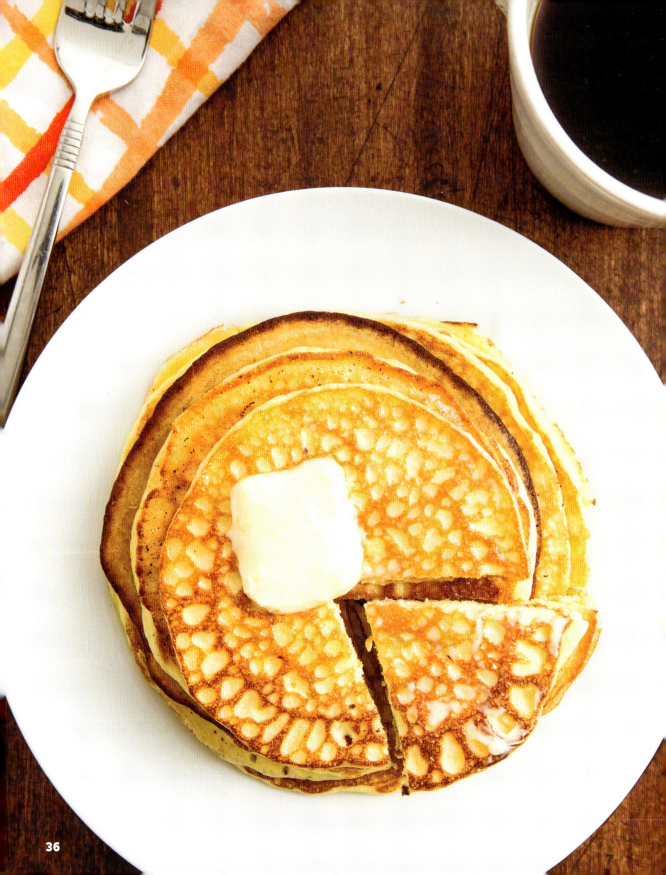

PERFECT PANCAKES

TOTAL TIME: 30 MIN / SERVES 5

You don't have to eat these plain: Toasted unsweetened coconut, a drizzle of melted peanut butter, a handful berries, or some crumbled bacon are all keto-friendly toppings.

½ cup almond flour

4 ounces cream cheese, softened

4 large eggs

1 teaspoon lemon zest

Butter, for frying and serving

1. In a medium bowl, whisk together almond flour, cream cheese, eggs, and lemon zest until smooth.

2. In a nonstick skillet over medium heat, melt 1 tablespoon butter. Pour in about 3 tablespoons batter and cook until golden, 2 minutes. Flip and cook 2 minutes more. Transfer to a plate and continue with the rest of the batter.

3. Serve topped with butter.

Nutrition (per serving): 110 calories, 4 g protein, 2 g carbohydrates, 1 g fiber, 1 g sugar, 10 g fat, 3.5 g saturated fat, 75 mg sodium

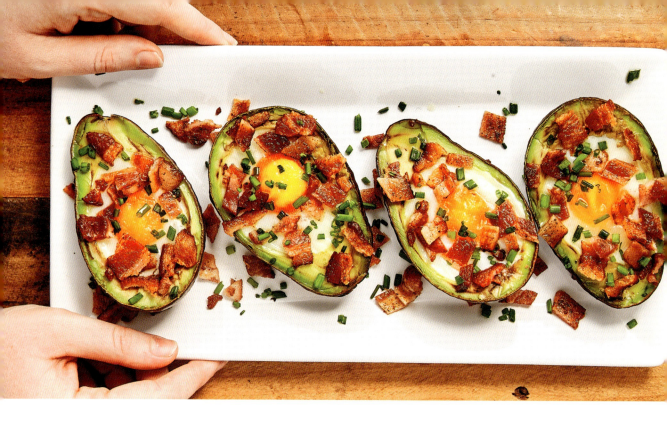

BAKED EGG AVOCADO BOATS

TOTAL TIME: 30 MIN / SERVES 4

Can't get enough avocado? Using the creamy fat as a baked egg boat is always a good idea.

2 ripe avocados, pitted and halved

4 large eggs

Kosher salt

Freshly ground black pepper

3 slices bacon

Freshly chopped chives, for garnish

1. Preheat oven to 350°. Place avocado halves in a baking dish, then crack eggs into a bowl. Using a spoon, transfer a yolk to each avocado half, then spoon in as much egg white as you can fit without spilling over.

2. Season with salt and pepper and bake until whites are set and yolks are no longer runny, about 20 minutes. (Cover with foil if avocados are beginning to brown.)

3. Meanwhile, in a large skillet over medium heat, cook bacon until crisp, 8 minutes, then transfer to a paper towel–lined plate and chop.

4. Top avocados with bacon and chives and serve with a spoon.

Nutrition (per serving): 220 calories, 10 g protein, 6 g carbohydrates, 5 g fiber, 0 g sugar, 18 g fat, 4 g saturated fat, 180 mg sodium

BREAKFAST WRAPS

TOTAL TIME: 15 MIN / SERVES 3

Everything you love about a breakfast wrap, minus the tortilla.

- 4 large eggs
- ¼ cup milk
- Kosher salt
- Freshly ground black pepper
- 1 tablespoon butter
- 1½ cups shredded cheddar, divided
- 6 breakfast sausages, cooked according to package instructions
- 1 avocado, cut into thin slices
- ½ cup grape tomatoes, quartered
- 1 tablespoon chopped chives for garnish

1. In a large bowl, whisk together eggs and milk. Season with salt and pepper.
2. In a medium skillet over medium heat, melt butter. Pour ⅓ of the egg mixture into the skillet, moving to create a thin layer that covers the entire pan.
3. Cook for 2 minutes. Add ½ cup cheddar and cover for 2 minutes more, until the cheese is melty.
4. Add sausage, avocado, and tomatoes to the center of egg wrap. Using a spatula, fold both ends over filling and "glue" shut with melted cheese. Remove from pan.
5. Garnish with chives and serve.

Nutrition (per serving): 720 calories, 34 g protein, 8 g carbohydrates, 3 g fiber, 3 g sugar, 60 g fat, 24 g saturated fat, 860 mg sodium

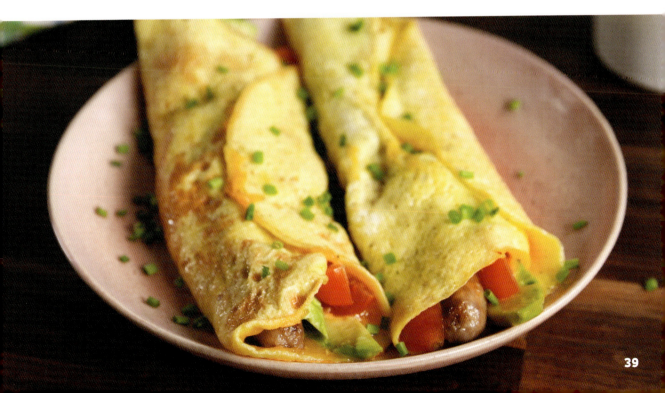

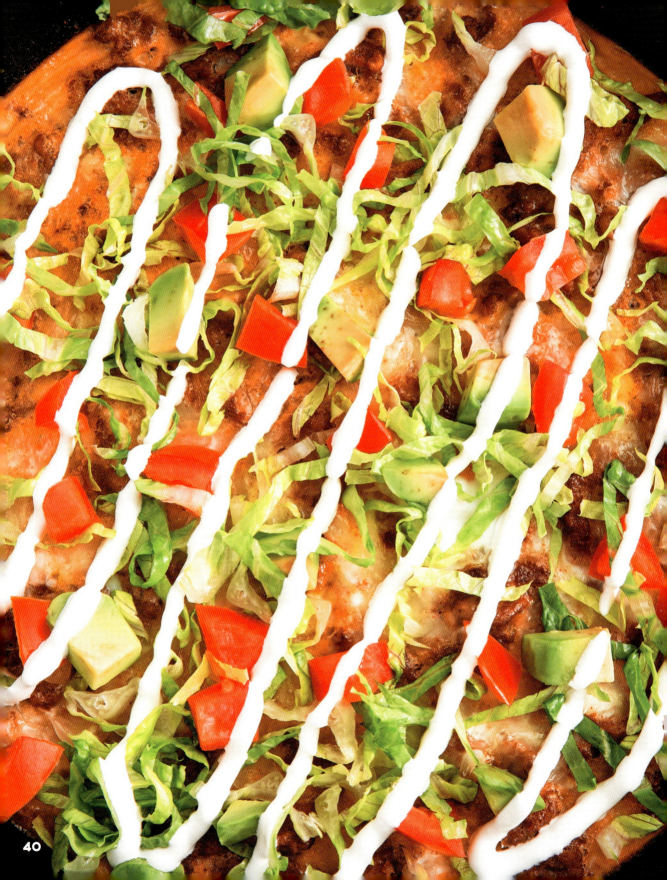

TACO BRUNCH CASSEROLE

TOTAL TIME: 50 MIN / SERVES 4

A fluffy egg and cheese layer tops seasoned ground meat in our brunch take on tacos.

1 tablespoon extra-virgin olive oil

1 pound ground turkey

1 tablespoon chili powder

1 teaspoon ground cumin

½ teaspoon garlic powder

Kosher salt

Freshly ground black pepper

Cooking spray

5 large eggs

½ cup whole milk

¾ cup shredded Monterey Jack

1 cup shredded romaine lettuce

1 medium tomato, chopped

1 small avocado, halved, pitted, and diced

Sour cream, for drizzling

1. Preheat oven to 350°. In a 10" ovenproof skillet over medium-high, heat oil.

2. Add ground turkey and season with chili powder, cumin, garlic powder, salt, and pepper. Cook, breaking up meat with back of a wooden spoon, until turkey is no longer pink, 6 to 8 minutes. Remove from heat and liberally coat the sides of the skillet with cooking spray.

3. In a medium bowl, whisk together eggs, milk, and cheese. Pour over the cooked ground turkey.

4. Bake until center of eggs are set, 30 to 40 minutes.

5. Garnish with lettuce, tomatoes, avocado, and sour cream before serving.

Nutrition (per serving): 360 calories, 15 g protein, 10 g carbohydrates, 3 g fiber, 3 g sugar, 22 g fat, 8 g saturated fat, 220 mg sodium

HAM & CHEESE EGG CUPS

TOTAL TIME: 35 MIN / SERVES 12

Our favorite way to use a muffin tin. These egg cups are totally adaptable: Swap out the cheddar for fontina or Gruyère and the ham for turkey or salami.

Cooking spray, for pan

12 slices ham

1 cup shredded cheddar

12 large eggs

Kosher salt

Freshly ground black pepper

Chopped fresh parsley, for garnish

1. Preheat oven to 400° and spray a 12-cup muffin tin with cooking spray.

2. Line each cup with a slice of ham and sprinkle with cheddar. Crack an egg in each ham cup and season with salt and pepper.

3. Bake until eggs are cooked through, 12 to 15 minutes (depending on how runny you like your yolks).

4. Garnish with parsley and serve.

Nutrition (per serving): 150 calories, 17 g protein, 1 g carbohydrates, 0 g fiber, 1 g sugar, 8 g fat, 3.5 g saturated fat, 740 mg sodium

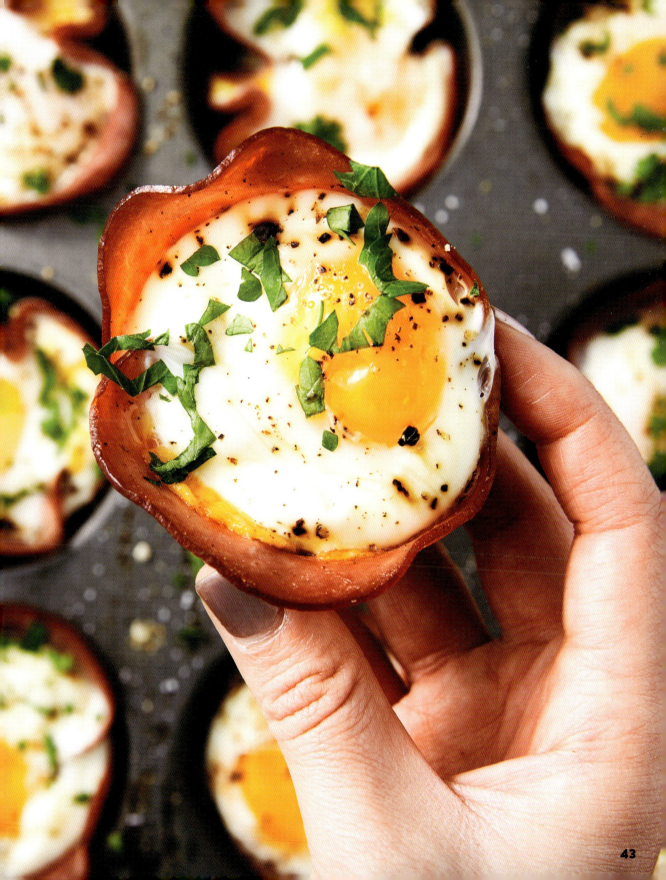

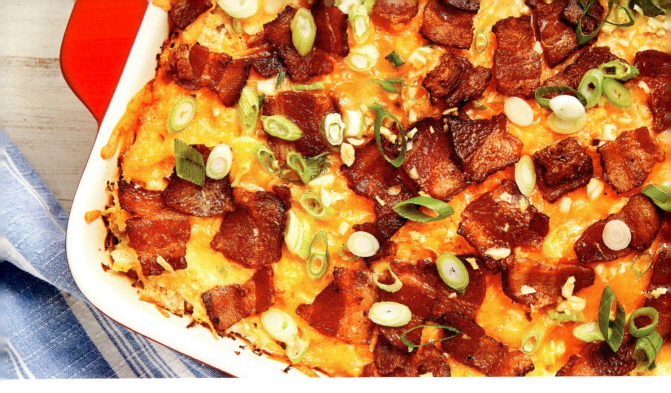

LOADED CAULIFLOWER BREAKFAST BAKE

TOTAL TIME: 55 MIN / SERVES 6

Ditch the hash browns for grated cauliflower and you'll have an extra-fluffy breakfast bake.

1 large head cauliflower
8 slices bacon, chopped
10 large eggs
1 cup whole milk
2 cloves garlic, minced
2 teaspoons paprika
Kosher salt
Freshly ground black pepper
2 cups shredded cheddar
2 green onions, thinly sliced, plus more for garnish
Hot sauce, for serving

1. Preheat oven to 350°. Grate cauliflower head on a box grater and transfer to a baking dish.
2. In a large skillet over medium heat, cook bacon. Transfer to a paper towel–lined plate to drain fat.
3. In a large bowl, whisk together eggs, milk, garlic, and paprika and season with salt and pepper.
4. Top cauliflower with cheddar, cooked bacon, and green onions, and pour over egg mixture.
5. Bake until eggs are set and top is golden, 35 to 40 minutes.
6. Garnish with green onions and more hot sauce and serve.

Nutrition (per serving): 390 calories, 28 g protein, 11 g carbohydrates, 3 g fiber, 5 g sugar, 27 g fat, 13 g saturated fat, 600 mg sodium

HAM, EGG & CHEESE ROLL-UPS

TOTAL TIME: 20 MIN / SERVES 5

Who needs a tortilla when you have sliced deli ham?
Make these in advance for an easy on-the-go breakfast.

- 10 large eggs
- 2 teaspoons garlic powder
- Kosher salt
- Freshly ground black pepper
- 2 tablespoons butter
- 1½ cups shredded cheddar
- 1 cup baby spinach
- 1 cup chopped tomatoes
- 20 slices ham

1. Heat broiler. In a large bowl, crack eggs. Whisk together with garlic powder and season with salt and pepper.

2. In a large nonstick skillet over medium heat, melt butter. Add eggs and scramble, stirring occasionally, 3 minutes. Stir in cheddar until melted, then stir in baby spinach and tomatoes until combined.

3. On a cutting board, place 2 slices of ham. Top with a big spoonful of scrambled eggs and roll up. Repeat with remaining ham and scrambled eggs.

4. Place roll-ups in a shallow baking dish and broil until ham is crispy, 5 minutes.

Nutrition (per serving): 410 calories, 38 g protein, 6 g carbohydrates, 1 g fiber, 4 g sugar, 26 g fat, 13 g saturated fat, 1620 mg sodium

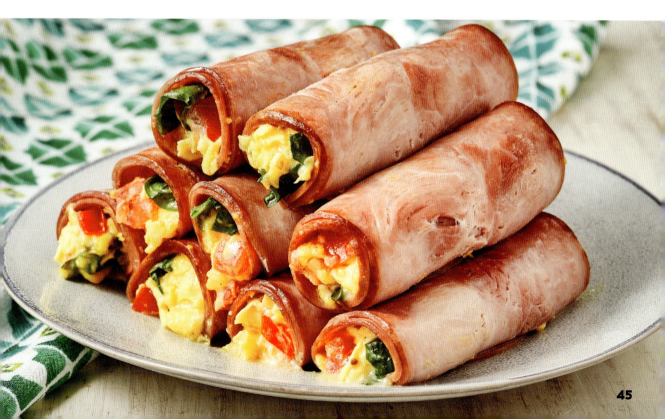

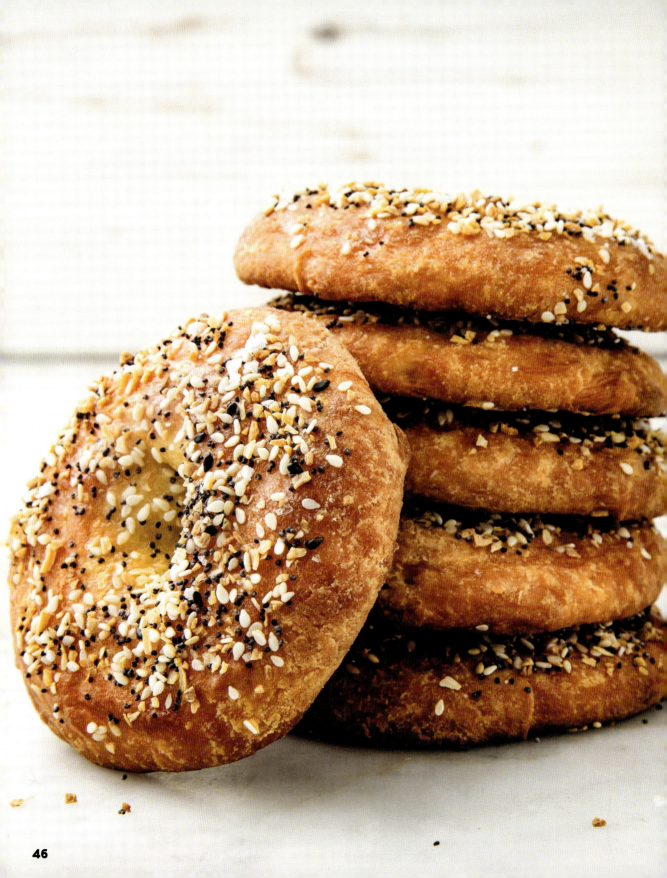

EVERYTHING KETO BAGELS

TOTAL TIME: 35 MIN / SERVES 8

Everyone should be able to enjoy a good bagel.
We love this version LOADED with everything seasoning.

2 cups almond flour

1 tablespoon baking powder

3 cups shredded mozzarella cheese

2 ounces cream cheese

2 large eggs, plus 1 large egg lightly beaten

3 tablespoons everything bagel seasoning

1. Preheat oven to 400°. Line 2 rimmed baking sheets with parchment paper. In a large bowl, whisk the almond flour with the baking powder. In a medium microwave-safe bowl, combine the mozzarella cheese and cream cheese. Microwave, stirring every 30 seconds, until the cheese is melted and combined, about 2 minutes total.

2. Scrape the cheese mixture into the bowl with the almond flour mixture and add the 2 eggs. Mix until well combined. Divide the dough into 8 equal portions. Roll each portion into a ball. Press your finger into the center of each ball and stretch to form a bagel shape. Arrange bagels on prepared baking sheets.

3. Brush the top of each bagel with beaten egg and sprinkle with everything bagel seasoning.

4. Bake on the middle rack for 20 to 24 minutes or until golden brown. Let cool 10 minutes before serving.

Nutrition (per serving): 359 calories, 19 g protein, 9 g carbohydrates, 3 g fiber, 2 g sugar, 29 g fat, 9 g saturated fat, 591 mg sodium

BACON WEAVE BREAKFAST TACOS

TOTAL TIME: 45 MIN / SERVES 4

Bacon in every. Single. Bite. Swapping tortillas for a bacon weave was possibly the smartest move ever.

16 slices bacon, halved

Freshly ground black pepper

6 large eggs

1 tablespoon whole milk

1 tablespoon unsalted butter

Kosher salt

2 tablespoons chopped chives

¼ cup shredded Monterey Jack

1 avocado, sliced

Hot sauce, for serving

1. Preheat oven to 400° and line a large, rimmed baking sheet with foil. In one corner, make a bacon weave with 8 halves of bacon, creating a square. Repeat to make next 3 weaves. Season with pepper. Place an inverted baking rack on top to make sure bacon lies flat.

2. Bake until bacon is crispy, 18 to 20 minutes. Working quickly, trim each square with a paring knife or kitchen shears to make a round shape.

3. Meanwhile, make scrambled eggs. In a medium bowl, whisk together eggs with milk until well incorporated.

4. In a medium, nonstick skillet over medium–low heat, melt butter. Pour egg mixture into the pan. Gently move the eggs around with a spatula, creating large curds. When the eggs are almost cooked to your liking, season with salt and pepper. Fold in chives and remove from heat.

5. Assemble tacos: On a serving platter, fill the bacon taco shells with scrambled eggs. Top each with cheese, a few slices of avocado, and top with hot sauce.

Nutrition (per serving): 390 calories, 24 g protein, 4 g carbohydrates, 2 g fiber, 1 g sugar, 31 g fat, 11 g saturated fat, 720 mg sodium

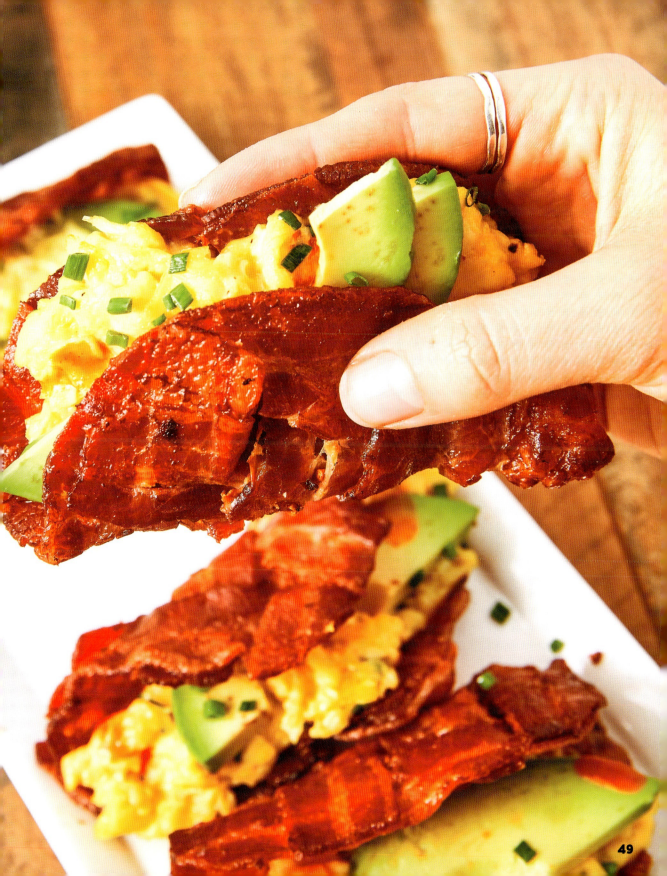

CAULI BREAKFAST HASH

TOTAL TIME: 50 MIN / SERVES 4 TO 6

Loaded with bell pepper, cheddar, and garlic, this cauli-hash totally beats potatoes.

6 slices bacon, cut into 1" pieces

1 onion, chopped

1 red bell pepper, chopped

1 large head cauliflower, chopped

Kosher salt

Freshly ground black pepper

¼ teaspoon smoked paprika

3 tablespoons water

2 cloves garlic, minced

2 tablespoons finely chopped chives

4 large eggs

1 cup shredded cheddar

1. In a large nonstick skillet over medium heat, fry bacon until crispy. Turn off heat and transfer bacon to a paper towel–lined plate. Keep most of bacon fat in skillet, removing any black pieces from the bottom.

2. Turn heat back to medium and add onion, bell pepper, and cauliflower to the skillet. Cook, stirring occasionally, until the vegetables begin to soften and turn golden, 5 to 8 minutes. Season with salt, pepper, and paprika.

3. Add 2 tablespoons of water and cover the skillet. Cook until the cauliflower is tender and the water has evaporated, about 5 minutes. (If all the water evaporates before the cauliflower is tender, add more water to the skillet and cover for a couple minutes more.)

4. Take off the lid, then stir in the garlic and chives and cook until the garlic is fragrant, about 30 seconds. Using a wooden spoon, make 4 holes in the hash to reveal bottom of skillet. Crack an egg into each hole and season each egg with salt and pepper. Sprinkle cheese and cooked bacon bits over the entire skillet. Replace lid and cook until eggs are cooked to your liking, about 5 minutes for a just-runny egg. Serve warm.

Nutrition (per serving): 220 calories, 15 g protein, 11 g carbohydrates, 4 g fiber, 5 g sugar, 13 g fat, 6 g saturated fat, 350 mg sodium

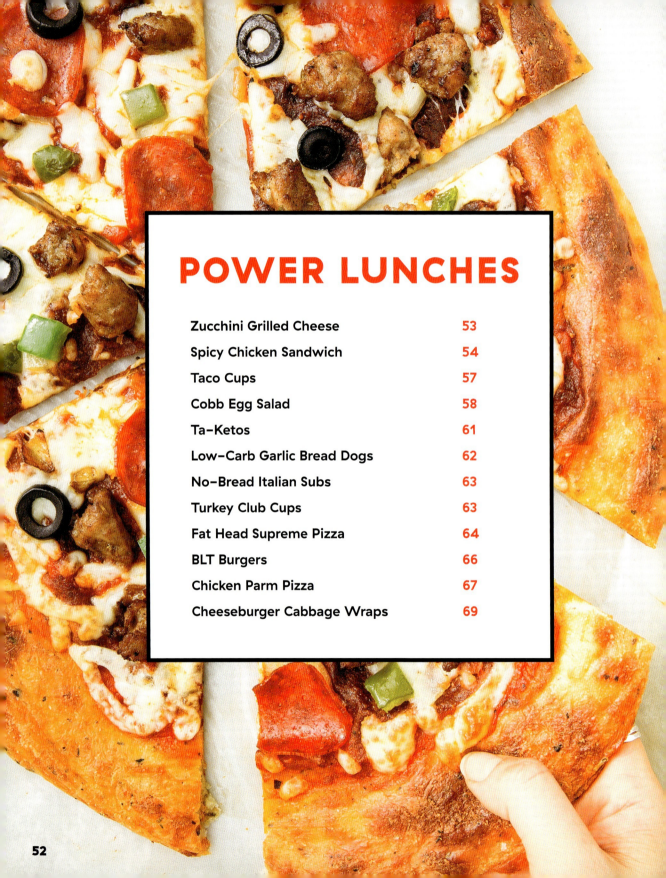

POWER LUNCHES

Zucchini Grilled Cheese	53
Spicy Chicken Sandwich	54
Taco Cups	57
Cobb Egg Salad	58
Ta-Ketos	61
Low-Carb Garlic Bread Dogs	62
No-Bread Italian Subs	63
Turkey Club Cups	63
Fat Head Supreme Pizza	64
BLT Burgers	66
Chicken Parm Pizza	67
Cheeseburger Cabbage Wraps	69

ZUCCHINI GRILLED CHEESE

TOTAL TIME: 40 MIN / SERVES 3 TO 4

Yeah, we went there: This grilled cheese has "bread" made out of grated zucchini. Pair it with your favorite low-carb tomato soup.

- 2 cups grated zucchini
- 1 large egg
- ½ cup freshly grated Parmesan
- 2 green onions, thinly sliced
- ¼ cup cornstarch
- Kosher salt
- Freshly ground black pepper
- Vegetable oil, for cooking
- 2 cups shredded cheddar

1. Squeeze excess moisture out of zucchini with a clean kitchen towel. In a medium bowl, combine zucchini with egg, Parmesan, green onions, and cornstarch. Season with salt and pepper.

2. In large skillet, pour enough vegetable oil to cover the bottom of the pan. Scoop about ¼ cup of the zucchini mixture onto one side of the pan and shape into a small square. Repeat to form another square on the other side.

3. Cook until lightly golden on both sides, about 4 minutes per side. Remove from heat to drain on paper towels and repeat with remaining zucchini mixture. Wipe skillet clean.

4. Place 2 zucchini patties in the same skillet over medium heat. Top both with shredded cheese, then place 2 more zucchini patties on top to form 2 sandwiches. Cook until the cheese has melted, about 2 minutes per side.

5. Repeat with remaining ingredients. Serve immediately.

Nutrition (per serving): 300 calories, 20 g protein, 4 g carbohydrates, 1 g fiber, 2 g sugar, 23 g fat, 14 g saturated fat, 530 mg sodium

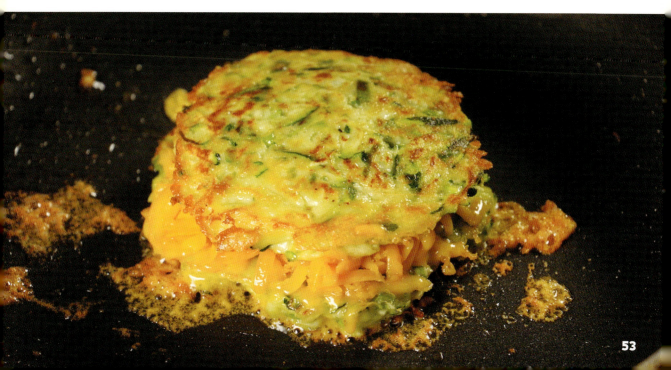

SPICY CHICKEN SANDWICH

TOTAL TIME: 30 MIN / SERVES 6

A chipotle-laced mayonnaise brings the heat to this killer chicken sandwich.

FOR THE BUNS:

2 cups shredded mozzarella

4 ounces cream cheese

3 large eggs

3 cups almond flour

2 teaspoons baking powder

1 teaspoon kosher salt

2 tablespoons butter, melted

FOR THE CHICKEN SANDWICH:

4 (6-ounce) boneless, skinless chicken breasts

Kosher salt

Freshly ground black pepper

2 tablespoons sweet paprika

1 tablespoon olive oil

2 tablespoons mayonnaise

1 tablespoon chopped chipotle chiles in adobo

½ avocado, halved, pitted, and sliced

2 tablespoons crumbled blue cheese

1 Preheat oven to 400° and line a baking sheet with parchment paper. In a large microwave-safe bowl, melt together mozzarella and cream cheese. Add eggs and stir to combine, then add almond flour, baking powder, and salt.

2 Form dough into 6 balls and flatten slightly, then place on prepared baking sheet. Brush with butter.

3 Bake until golden, 10 to 12 minutes. Let cool slightly.

4 Season chicken breasts with salt, pepper, and paprika. In a large skillet over medium-high heat, heat oil. Cook chicken until golden on both sides, 8 minutes per side.

5 In a small bowl, mix mayo and chipotle chiles until combined.

6 To assemble the sandwiches, thinly slice chicken. Halve buns and spread chipotle mayonnaise on each side. Top with chicken slices, avocado, and blue cheese. Top with bun half and serve.

Nutrition (per serving): 720 calories, 42 g protein, 16 g carbohydrates, 7 g fiber, 3 g sugar, 57 g fat, 15 g saturated fat, 1040 mg sodium

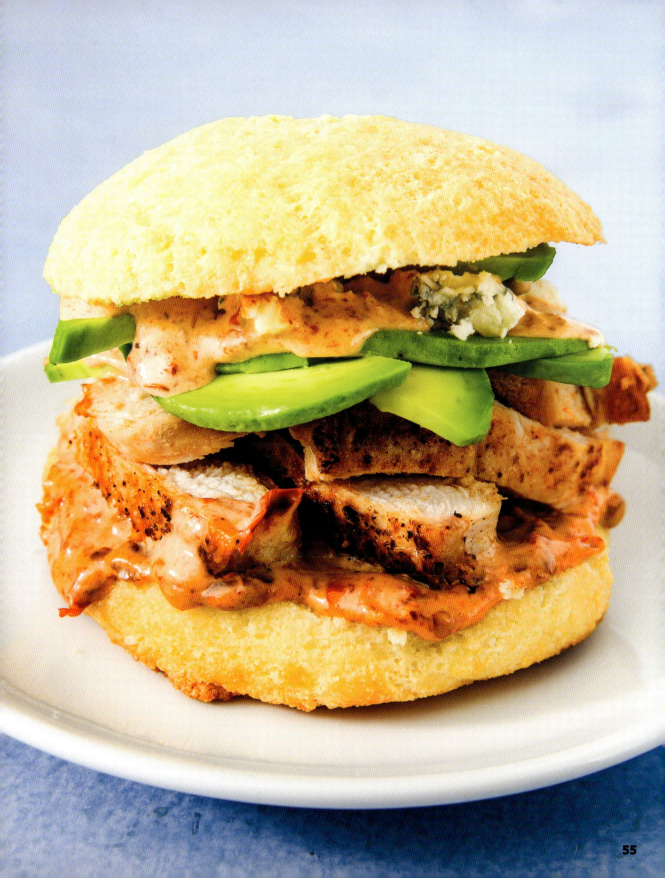

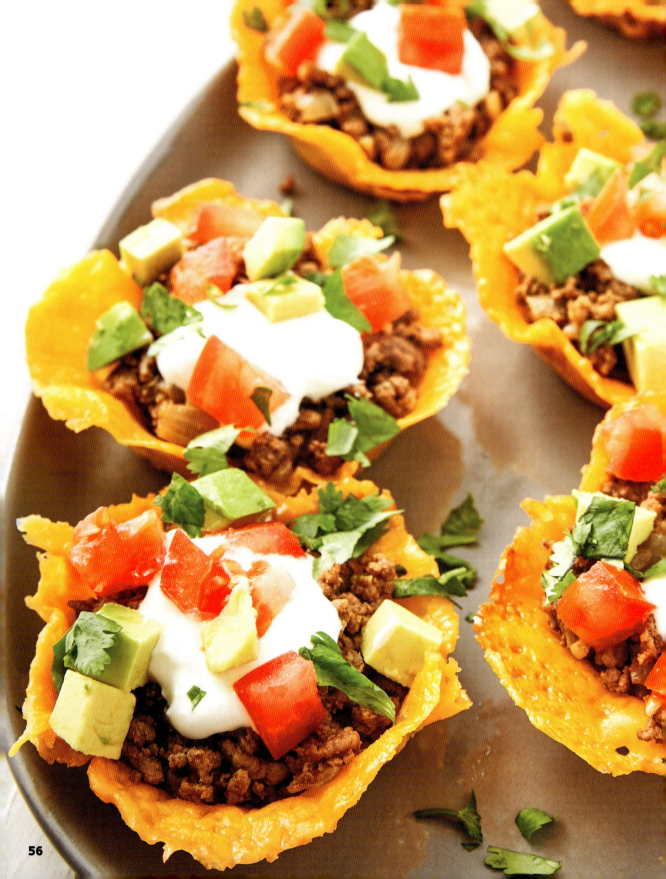

TACO CUPS

TOTAL TIME: 30 MIN / SERVES 8

No tortillas, no problem. With your muffin tin, you can turn shredded cheddar into serving cups.

3½ cups shredded cheddar

Cooking spray

1 tablespoon extra-virgin olive oil

1 onion, chopped

3 cloves garlic, minced

1 pound ground beef

1 teaspoon chili powder

½ teaspoon ground cumin

½ teaspoon paprika

Kosher salt

Freshly ground black pepper

Sour cream, for serving

Diced avocado, for serving

Chopped cilantro, for serving

Chopped tomatoes, for serving

1 Preheat oven to 375° and line a large baking sheet with parchment paper. Spoon about a tablespoon of cheese at a time, a few inches apart. Bake until bubbly and edges are beginning to turn golden, about 6 minutes. Let cool on baking sheet for a minute.

2 Meanwhile, grease bottom of a muffin tin with cooking spray, then carefully pick up melted cheese slices and place on bottom of muffin tin. Let cool 10 minutes.

3 In a large skillet over medium heat, heat olive oil. Add onion and cook, stirring occasionally, until soft, about 5 minutes. Stir in garlic, then add ground beef, breaking up the meat with a wooden spoon. Cook until beef is no longer pink, about 6 minutes, then drain fat. Season with chili powder, cumin, paprika, salt, and pepper.

4 Transfer cheese cups to a serving platter. Fill with cooked ground beef, then top with sour cream, avocado, cilantro, and tomatoes.

Nutrition (per serving): 300 calories, 25 g protein, 2 g carbohydrates, 0 g fiber, 1 g sugar, 21 g fat, 12 g saturated fat, 350 mg sodium

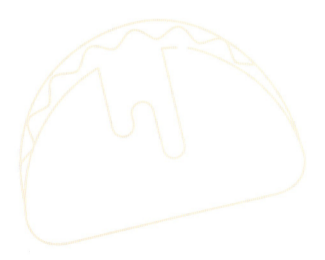

COBB EGG SALAD

TOTAL TIME: 20 MIN / SERVES 6

Sure, egg salad is great. But an egg salad with bacon, blue cheese, and avocado? Now that's a lunch you'll be dreaming about for days.

FOR THE DRESSING:

3 tablespoons mayonnaise

3 tablespoons Greek yogurt

2 tablespoons red wine vinegar

Kosher salt

Freshly ground black pepper

FOR THE SALAD:

8 large hard-boiled eggs, cut into 8 pieces, plus more for garnish

8 strips bacon, cooked and crumbled, plus more for garnish

1 avocado, thinly sliced

½ cup crumbled blue cheese, plus more for garnish

½ cup cherry tomatoes, halved, plus more for garnish

2 tablespoons freshly chopped chives

1 In a small bowl, stir together mayonnaise, yogurt, and red wine vinegar. Season with salt and pepper.

2 In a large serving bowl, gently mix together eggs, bacon, avocado, blue cheese, and cherry tomatoes. Gradually fold in mayonnaise dressing, using only enough until ingredients are lightly coated, then season with salt and pepper. Garnish with chives and additional toppings.

Nutrition (per serving): 336 calories, 18 g protein, 5 g carbohydrates, 2 g fiber, 2 g sugar, 27 g fat, 8 g saturated fat, 655 mg sodium

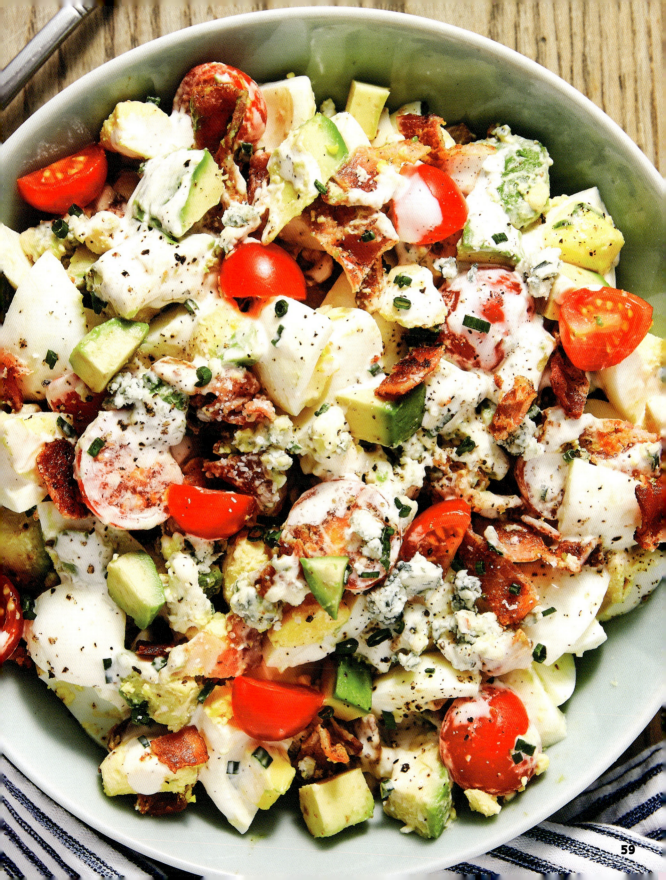

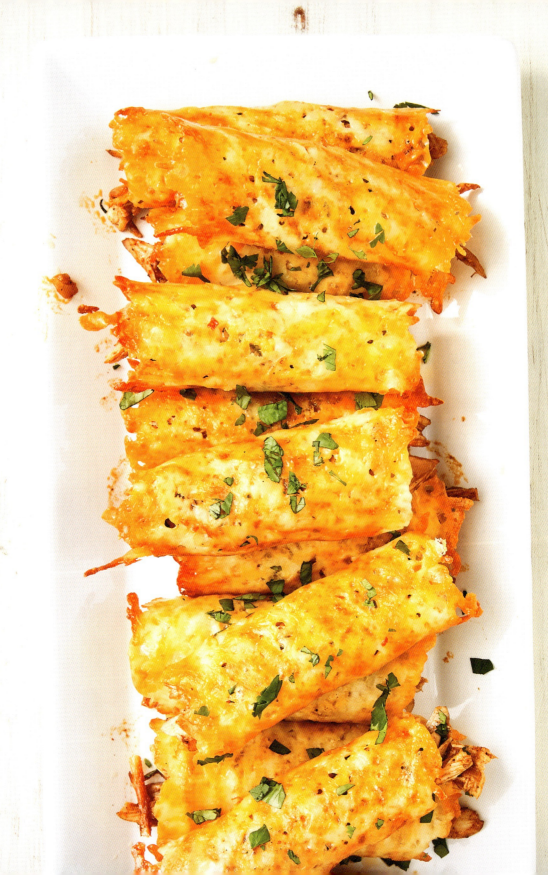

TA-KETOS

TOTAL TIME: 20 MIN / SERVES 6

These might sound tricky, but they're surprisingly easy to make.
Just make sure to roll them up while the cheese is still warm.

1 tablespoon extra-virgin olive oil
¼ onion, finely chopped
2 garlic cloves, minced
½ teaspoon cumin
½ teaspoon chili powder
1½ cups shredded chicken
⅓ cup red enchilada sauce
2 tablespoons freshly chopped cilantro, plus more for garnish
Kosher salt
1 cup shredded cheddar
1 cup shredded Monterey Jack
Sour cream, for serving (optional)

1 Preheat oven to 375° and line a small baking sheet with parchment paper. In a medium skillet over medium heat, heat oil. Add onion and cook until slightly soft, 3 minutes. Add garlic and spices and cook until fragrant, 1 to 2 minutes more.

2 Add chicken and enchilada sauce, then bring mixture to a simmer. Stir in cilantro, season with salt, and remove from heat.

3 Make shells: In a medium bowl, mix together cheeses. Divide mixture into 6 piles on prepared baking sheet. Bake 8 to 10 minutes, or until cheese is melted and slightly golden around the edges. Let cool 2 to 4 minutes, then add a small pile of chicken and roll tightly. Repeat until all shells are filled.

4 Garnish with cilantro and serve with sour cream, for dipping.

Nutrition (per serving): 230 calories, 17 g protein, 2 g carbohydrates, 0 g fiber, 0 g sugar, 18 g fat, 9 g saturated fat, 310 mg sodium

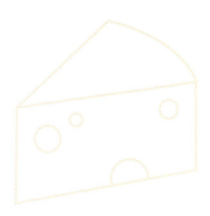

LOW-CARB GARLIC BREAD DOGS

TOTAL TIME: 25 MIN / SERVES 6

We swapped out the traditional hot dog bun for an easy-to-make keto bread that wraps around the dog.

- 2 cups shredded mozzarella
- 4 ounces cream cheese
- 2 large eggs, beaten
- 2½ cups almond flour
- 2 teaspoons baking powder
- 1 teaspoon kosher salt
- 8 hot dogs, such as Applegate Natural Beef Hot Dogs
- 4 tablespoons butter, melted
- 1 teaspoon garlic powder
- 1 tablespoon freshly chopped parsley
- Mustard, for serving

1. Preheat oven to 400° and line a baking sheet with parchment paper. In a large microwave-safe bowl, combine mozzarella and cream cheese and microwave until melty, about 1 minute.

2. Add eggs and stir to combine then add almond flour, baking powder, and salt.

3. Divide dough into 8 balls then shape each ball into long ropes then wrap a rope around each hot dog.

4. In a small bowl whisk together butter, garlic powder, and parsley. Brush garlic butter over each hot dog then bake until golden, 10 to 15 minutes.

5. Serve with mustard, for dipping.

Nutrition (per serving): 590 calories, 28 g protein, 13 g carbohydrates, 5 g fiber, 3 g sugar, 49 g fat, 17 g saturated fat, 1430 mg sodium

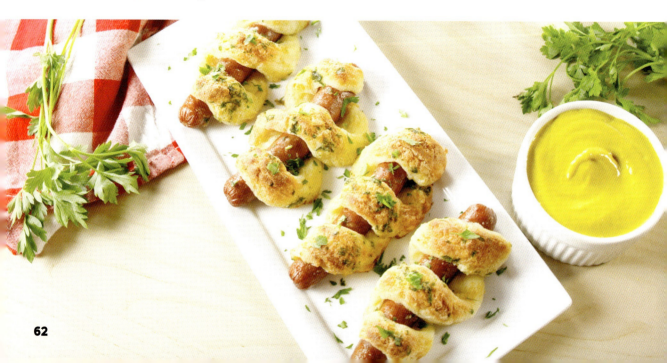

NO-BREAD ITALIAN SUBS

TOTAL TIME: 15 MIN / SERVES 6

No hoagie roll, no prob. These Italian sub roll-ups include only the best part of the sandwich.

½ cup mayonnaise

2 tablespoons red wine vinegar

1 tablespoon extra-virgin olive oil

1 small garlic clove, grated

1 teaspoon Italian seasoning

6 slices ham

12 slices salami

12 slices pepperoni

6 slices provolone

1 cup shredded romaine

½ cup roasted red peppers

1 Make creamy Italian dressing: In a small bowl, whisk together mayo, vinegar, oil, garlic, and Italian seasoning until emulsified.

2 Assemble sandwiches: Layer a slice of ham, two slices salami, two slices pepperoni, and a slice of provolone.

3 Add a handful of lettuce and a few roasted red peppers in the middle. Drizzle with creamy Italian dressing, then roll up to serve. Repeat with remaining ingredients until you have 6 roll-ups.

Nutrition (per serving): 390 calories, 16 g protein, 3 g carbohydrates, 0 g fiber, 1 g sugar, 34 g fat, 10 g saturated fat, 1210 mg sodium

TURKEY CLUB CUPS

TOTAL TIME: 20 MIN / SERVES 12

The classic sandwich becomes an even easier-to-eat finger food.

Cooking spray

12 slices roasted deli turkey

12 slices sharp cheddar

¼ cup mayonnaise

2 tablespoons Dijon mustard

½ head iceberg lettuce, shredded

1 pint cherry tomatoes, chopped

1 avocado, halved, pitted and chopped

8 slices bacon, cooked and chopped

1 Preheat oven to 400° and lightly grease muffin tin with cooking spray.

2 Place a slice of turkey into each muffin cup. Add a slice of cheddar, then bake until turkey is sturdy and cheese is melted, about 10 minutes. Let cool slightly.

3 Meanwhile, in a small bowl, mix together mayo and Dijon. Add a dollop to the bottom of each turkey cup and spread around. Fill with lettuce, cherry tomatoes, avocado, and bacon.

4 Repeat to fill cups.

Nutrition (per serving): 230 calories, 17 g protein, 5 g carbohydrates, 1 g fiber, 1 g sugar, 16 g fat, 6 g saturated fat, 800 mg sodium

FAT HEAD SUPREME PIZZA

TOTAL TIME: 30 MIN / SERVES 4

"Fat Head" crust is blowing up on Pinterest. The combo of almond flour, mozzarella, and egg tastes bizarrely similiar to the real thing.

FOR THE TOPPINGS:

½ tablespoon extra-virgin olive oil

½ onion, chopped

1 bell pepper, chopped

2 Italian sausage links, removed from casings

⅓ cup marinara sauce

3 tablespoons shredded mozzarella

¼ cup sliced black olives

8 slices pepperoni

FOR THE PIZZA CRUST:

2 cups shredded mozzarella

2 ounces cream cheese

⅔ cup almond flour

1 large egg

1 teaspoon Italian seasoning

1 Preheat the oven to 425° and line a large baking sheet with parchment paper. In a small skillet over medium-high heat, heat oil. Add onion and bell pepper and cook 4 minutes. Add sausage and cook, breaking up meat with a wooden spoon, until seared and no longer pink, about 5 minutes.

2 Make pizza crust: In a medium microwave-safe bowl, combine 2 cups shredded mozzarella and cream cheese and microwave until melty, about 1 minute. Stir in almond flour, egg, and Italian seasoning until fully combined.

3 Place pizza dough on prepared baking sheet. Using wet hands, spread the dough into an oval shape as thin as dough will allow. Bake 10 minutes.

4 Use a fork to poke holes in the dough if it has puffed up. Spread marinara sauce over crust and top with 3 tablespoons mozzarella, sausage mixture, olives, and pepperoni.

5 Bake until cheese is melty, 4 to 6 minutes. Let cool slightly before slicing into 8 pieces.

Nutrition (per serving): 550 calories, 30 g protein, 13 g carbohydrates, 3 g fiber, 3 g sugar, 42 g fat, 15 g saturated fat, 1100 mg sodium

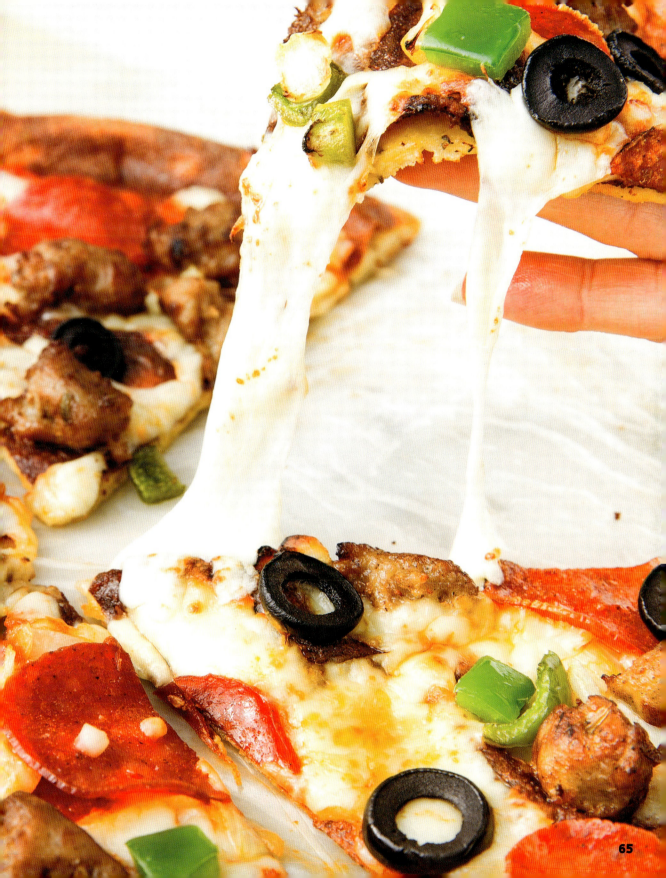

BLT BURGERS

TOTAL TIME: 35 MIN / SERVES 4

Everything, even a burger, is better with a bacon weave bun.
Don't even think about skipping the herb mayo.

1 pound bacon slices, halved

Freshly ground black pepper

1 pound ground beef

Kosher salt

½ cup mayonnaise

Juice of ½ lemon

3 tablespoons finely chopped chives

Butterhead lettuce, for serving

2 tomatoes, sliced

1. Preheat oven to 400° and place a baking rack inside of a baking sheet (to help catch grease).

2. Make a bacon weave: On the baking rack, line 3 bacon halves side-by-side. Lift one end of the middle bacon slice and place a 4th bacon half on top of the side pieces and underneath the middle slice. Lay the middle slice back down.

3. Next, lift the 2 side strips of bacon and place a 5th bacon half on top of the middle piece and underneath the sides. Lay the side slices back down.

4. Finally, lift the other end of the middle slice and place a 6th slice on top of the side pieces and underneath the middle slice. Repeat to make a second weave.

5. Season with pepper and bake until bacon is crispy, 25 minutes. Transfer to a paper towel–lined plate to blot grease. Let cool for at least 10 minutes.

6. Meanwhile, make burgers: Preheat a grill (or grill pan) to medium-high heat. Shape ground beef into large patties and season both sides with salt and pepper. Grill until cooked to your liking, about 4 minutes per side for medium.

7. Make herb mayo: In a small bowl, whisk together mayonnaise, lemon juice, and chives.

8. Assemble burgers: For each burger, place a bacon weave on the bottom then spread it with some herb mayo. Top with burger, lettuce, tomato, and another bacon weave. Serve immediately.

Nutrition (per serving): 980 calories, 67 g protein, 4 g carbohydrates, 1 g fiber, 2 g sugar, 75 g fat, 21 g saturated fat, 2180 mg sodium

CHICKEN PARM PIZZA

TOTAL TIME: 40 MIN / SERVES 4

Not getting enough color on your chicken "crust?" Try broiling it for a few minutes to get it extra golden.

- 1 pound ground chicken
- ¾ cup freshly grated Parmesan, divided
- ½ teaspoon Italian seasoning
- 1 garlic clove, minced
- Kosher salt
- Freshly ground black pepper
- Cooking spray
- ¼ cup marinara sauce
- ½ cup freshly shredded mozzarella
- Red pepper flakes, for serving (optional)
- Basil leaves, for garnish

1. Preheat oven to 400° and line a large baking sheet with parchment paper. In a large bowl, stir together ground chicken, ½ cup Parmesan, Italian seasoning, and garlic. Season with salt and pepper.

2. Spray prepared baking sheet with cooking spray. Form chicken mixture into a large round crust, about ½" thick.

3. Bake until chicken is cooked through and golden, 20 to 22 minutes. Remove from oven and preheat the broiler.

4. Spread a thin layer of marinara sauce, leaving a small border around the circumference of the pizza. Top with mozzarella and broil until cheese is melty, 3 to 4 minutes. Garnish with remaining ¼ cup Parmesan, red pepper flakes if using, and fresh basil.

Nutrition (per serving): 270 calories, 30 g protein, 2 g carbohydrates, 0 g fiber, 1 g sugar, 17 g fat, 7 g saturated fat, 400 mg sodium

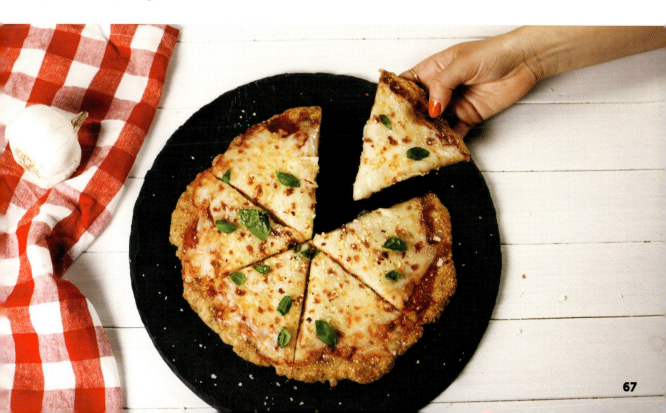

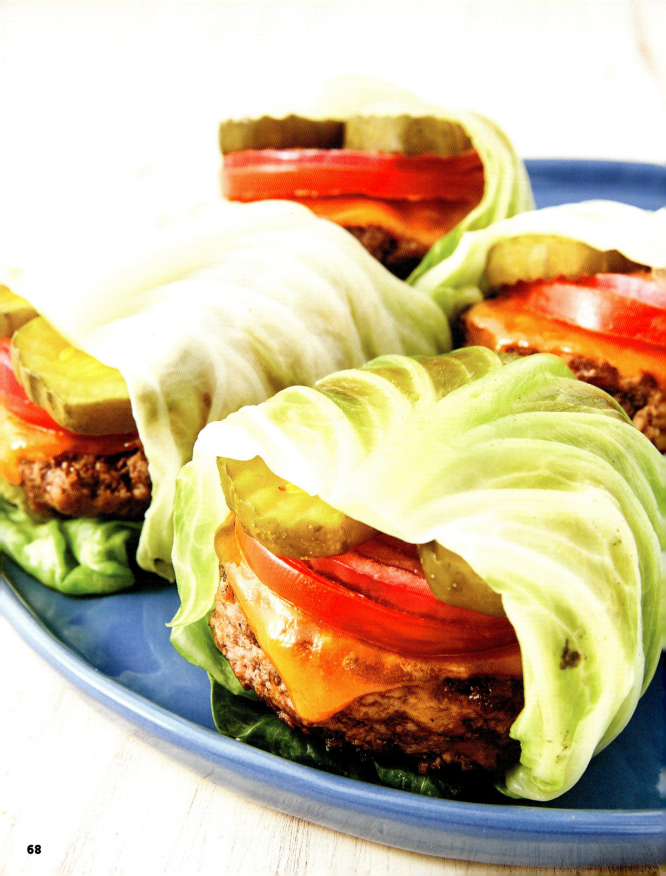

CHEESEBURGER CABBAGE WRAPS

TOTAL TIME: 55 MIN / SERVES 4

Who needs a burger bun? We love how sturdy cabbage is as a bun replacement—just make sure you buy a large cabbage so your leaves are big enough to wrap around the entire burger.

FOR THE CABBAGE WRAPS:

4 large green cabbage leaves (from 1 head)

1 pound ground beef

Kosher salt

Freshly ground black pepper

4 slices cheddar cheese

½ red onion, thinly sliced into rounds

1 medium tomato, sliced

Pickle chips, for serving

FOR THE SAUCE:

2 tablespoons mayonnaise

2 tablespoons Dijon mustard

1 teaspoon red wine vinegar

½ teaspoon garlic powder

Kosher salt

Freshly ground black pepper

1 In a large pot of boiling water, use tongs to dip cabbage leaves in water for 30 seconds to blanch. Place on a paper towel–lined plate to dry.

2 Make sauce: In a medium bowl, combine mayonnaise, mustard, vinegar, and garlic powder. Season with salt and pepper and whisk until smooth.

3 Make burgers: Form ground beef into 4 patties; season both sides with salt and pepper. Heat a large skillet over medium-high heat. Add patties and cook until burgers are seared on the bottom, 4 to 6 minutes. Flip burgers and cook until cooked through to your liking (4 to 6 minutes for medium), adding cheese during the last minute of cooking.

4 Assemble burgers: Place burger patty on the edge of a cabbage leaf where the thickest part of the stem is. Top with onion, tomato, and pickles. Fold opposite end of cabbage leaf up over burger, then fold one side of cabbage leaf over burger and roll until burger is completely wrapped. Serve with sauce.

Nutrition (per serving): 383 calories, 29 g protein, 6 g carbohydrates, 2 g fiber, 3 g sugar, 27 g fat, 11 g saturated fat, 834 mg sodium

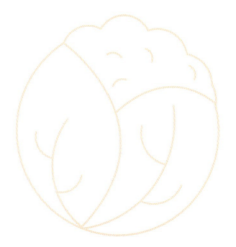

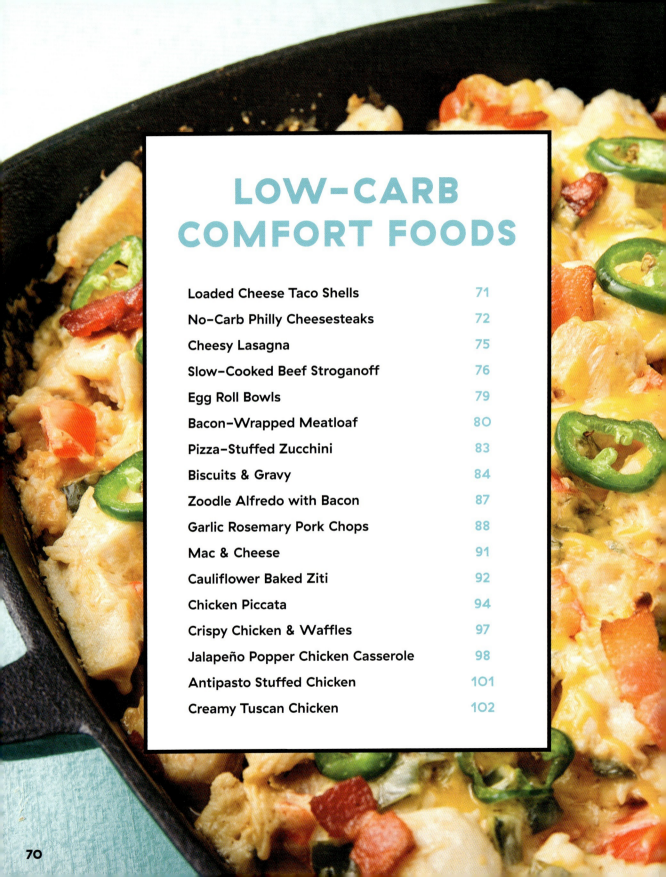

LOW-CARB COMFORT FOODS

Loaded Cheese Taco Shells	71
No-Carb Philly Cheesesteaks	72
Cheesy Lasagna	75
Slow-Cooked Beef Stroganoff	76
Egg Roll Bowls	79
Bacon-Wrapped Meatloaf	80
Pizza-Stuffed Zucchini	83
Biscuits & Gravy	84
Zoodle Alfredo with Bacon	87
Garlic Rosemary Pork Chops	88
Mac & Cheese	91
Cauliflower Baked Ziti	92
Chicken Piccata	94
Crispy Chicken & Waffles	97
Jalapeño Popper Chicken Casserole	98
Antipasto Stuffed Chicken	101
Creamy Tuscan Chicken	102

LOADED CHEESE TACO SHELLS

TOTAL TIME: 30 MIN / SERVES 4

When you make your shell out of cheddar, Taco Tuesday can totally still happen on keto. These deliver on crunch and flavor.

Cooking spray

2 cups shredded cheddar

Freshly ground black pepper

1 tablespoon vegetable oil

1 white onion, chopped

1 pound ground beef

1 tablespoon taco seasoning

Shredded lettuce, for serving

Chopped tomatoes, for serving

Hot sauce, for serving

1. Preheat oven to 375°. Line a baking sheet with parchment paper and spray with cooking spray. Place ½-cup mounds of cheddar on baking sheet and season with pepper.

2. Bake until cheese is melty and slightly crispy, 5 to 7 minutes. Blot grease with a paper towel.

3. Meanwhile, set up 4 stations of 2 upside-down glasses and a wooden spoon as a bridge. Using a spatula, immediately transfer cheese mounds to wooden spoons to form shells. Let cool.

4. Meanwhile, make taco meat: In a large skillet over medium heat, heat oil. Add onions and cook until soft, 5 minutes, then add ground beef and cook until no longer pink, 6 minutes more. Drain fat and season with taco seasoning.

5. Assemble tacos: Place beef in shells and top with lettuce, tomatoes, and hot sauce.

Nutrition (per serving): 430 calories, 39 g protein, 4 g carbohydrates, 1 g fiber, 2 g sugar, 28 g fat, 16 g saturated fat, 480 mg sodium

NO-CARB PHILLY CHEESESTEAKS

TOTAL TIME: 30 MIN / SERVES 4

All the ingredients you love in the classic sandwich—
steak, peppers, onions, provolone—all loaded in a lettuce wrap.

2 tablespoons vegetable oil, divided

1 large onion, thinly sliced

2 large bell peppers, thinly sliced

1 teaspoon dried oregano

Kosher salt

Freshly ground black pepper

1 pound skirt steak, thinly sliced

1 cup shredded provolone

8 large butterhead lettuce leaves

1 tablespoon chopped parsley for garnish

1. Heat 1 tablespoon of oil in a large skillet over medium heat, then add onion and bell peppers. Season with oregano, salt and pepper. Cook, stirring often, until the onions and peppers are tender, about 5 minutes. Remove peppers and onions from skillet and heat remaining 1 tablespoon oil in skillet.

2. Add steak slices in a single layer and season with salt and pepper. Sear steak on one side, about 2 minutes. Flip and cook until the steak is seared on the second side and is done to your liking, about 2 minutes more for medium.

3. Add onion mixture back to skillet and toss to combine. Sprinkle provolone over steak and onions then cover skillet with a tight-fitting lid and cook until the cheese has melted, about 1 minute. Remove from heat.

4. Arrange lettuce on a serving platter. Scoop $\frac{1}{8}$ of the steak mixture onto each piece of lettuce. Garnish with parsley and serve warm.

Nutrition (per serving): 370 calories, 31 g protein, 7 g carbohydrates, 2 g fiber, 3 g sugar, 23 g fat, 9 g saturated fat, 250 mg sodium

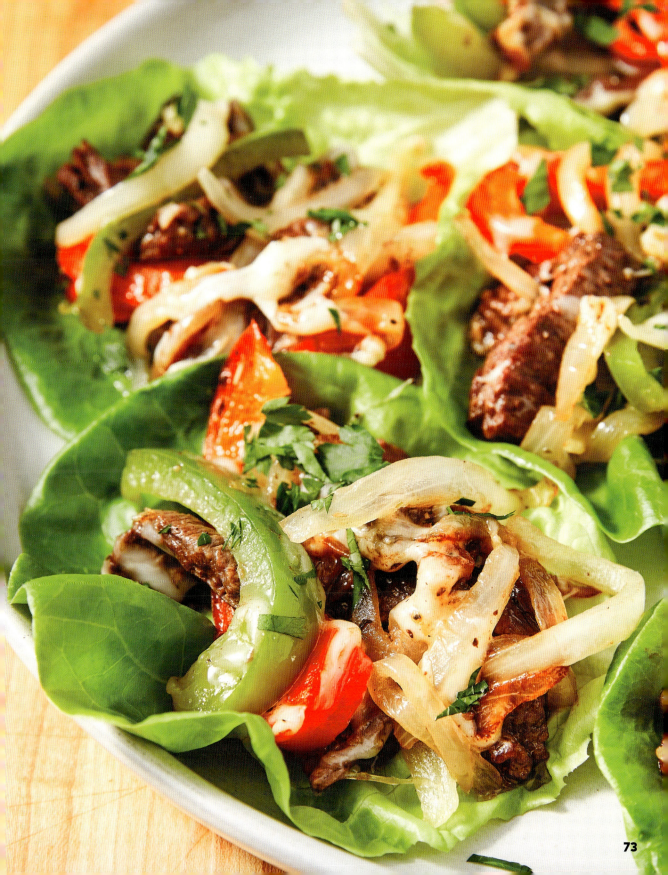

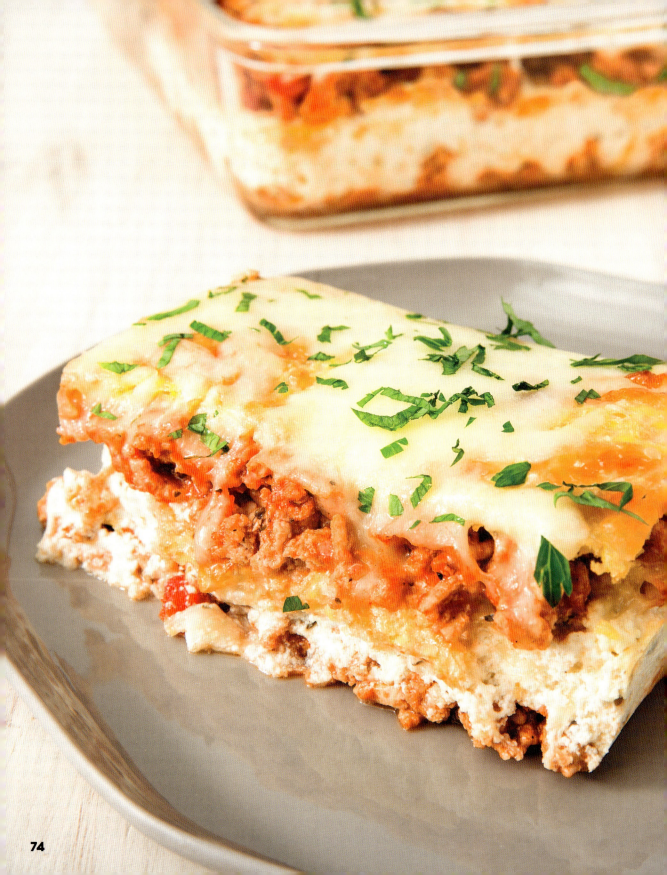

CHEESY LASAGNA

TOTAL TIME: 1 HR / SERVES 8

Packaged cauliflower rice makes this noodle-free lasagna a cinch to pull off.

FOR THE "NOODLE" LAYER:

3 large eggs

1 (12-ounce) container riced cauliflower (about 2½ cups)

1 cup shredded mozzarella

Kosher salt

FOR THE MEAT FILLING:

½ tablespoon extra-virgin olive oil

1 pound ground turkey

1 teaspoon Italian seasoning

Kosher salt

Freshly ground black pepper

2 tablespoons tomato paste

¾ cup crushed tomatoes

FOR THE CHEESE FILLING:

1 cup ricotta cheese

¾ cup shredded mozzarella, divided

¼ cup grated Parmesan

1 large egg, beaten

1 teaspoon Italian seasoning

Kosher salt

Freshly ground black pepper

Freshly chopped parsley, for garnish

1. Preheat the oven to 350° and line a rimmed half sheet pan with parchment paper. In a large bowl, beat eggs, then stir in cauliflower, 1 cup mozzarella, and salt. Spread cauliflower mixture onto prepared sheet pan in an even layer about ¾-inch thick.

2. Bake until firm to the touch and golden, 25 minutes. Let cool 10 minutes, and increase oven temperature to 400°.

3. Meanwhile, in a medium skillet over medium-high heat, heat oil. Add ground turkey and season with Italian seasoning, salt, and pepper. Cook turkey, breaking up the meat with back of a wooden spoon, until no longer pink, 6 to 8 minutes. Stir in tomato paste and crushed tomatoes and cook 2 minutes, stirring constantly. Remove from heat.

4. In a medium bowl, mix ricotta cheese, ½ cup mozzarella, Parmesan, egg, and Italian seasoning until combined. Season with salt and pepper.

5. Grease an 8"-x-8" baking dish with cooking spray. Add half the meat to the baking pan. Cut the cauliflower "noodle" layer into strips and place in baking dish to fit bottom layer. Top with entire ricotta mixture and more cauliflower noodles, then top with remaining meat and cauliflower noodles. Sprinkle remaining ¼ cup shredded mozzarella on top.

6. Bake in oven until golden, 20 to 25 minutes.

7. Garnish with parsley before serving.

Nutrition (per serving): 250 calories, 29 g protein, 7 g carbohydrates, 2 g fiber, 3 g sugar, 13 g fat, 6 g saturated fat, 380 mg sodium

SLOW-COOKED BEEF STROGANOFF

TOTAL TIME: 4½ HR OR 8½ HR / SERVES 4

Fork-tender chunks of beef slowly cook with meaty mushrooms for a keto-friendly stroganoff. The mushrooms give off liquid as they soften, which means less broth is needed at the beginning.

2 pounds top round beef roast, cut into 1" pieces

Kosher salt

Freshly ground black pepper

2 tablespoons extra-virgin olive oil

1 (16-ounce) package sliced mushrooms, finely chopped

½ cup low-sodium beef broth

2 cloves garlic, minced

2 teaspoons low-sodium soy sauce

8 cups chopped cauliflower florets (from about 1 large head)

⅓ cup milk, plus more if needed

1 tablespoon butter

⅓ cup sour cream

½ cup freshly chopped parsley, for garnish

1. Season beef with salt and pepper. In a large skillet over medium-high heat, heat oil. Add beef and cook until seared, 3 minutes per side.

2. Transfer beef to bowl of a large slow cooker then add mushrooms, beef broth, garlic, and soy sauce. Season with salt and pepper.

3. Cover with lid and cook until the beef is fork-tender, 4 hours on high or 8 hours on low. Turn off heat. Drain some of the liquid, if needed. Stir in sour cream and season with salt and pepper.

4. When beef is almost done, fill a large pot with 3" of water and add a steamer insert. Bring water to a boil over high heat then add cauliflower and cover with lid. Steam until fork-tender, 12 to 15 minutes.

5. Carefully transfer cauliflower to the bowl of a food processor. Add milk and butter and season with salt and pepper. Pulse until smooth, adding a little more milk if needed.

6. Serve stroganoff over cauliflower and garnish with parsley.

Nutrition (per serving): 390 calories, 40 g protein, 11 g carbohydrates, 4 g fiber, 5 g sugar, 21 g fat, 8 g saturated fat, 230 mg sodium

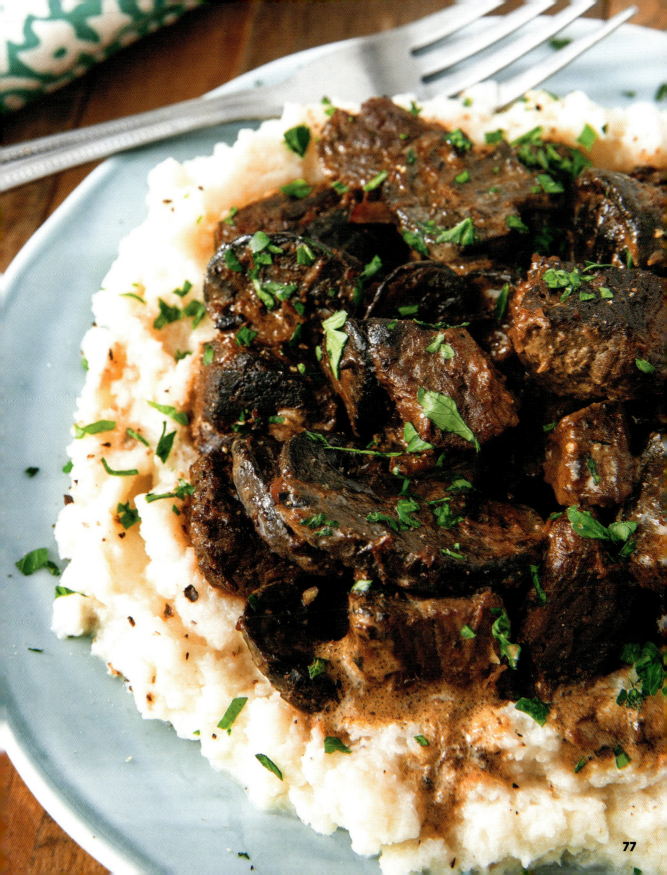

77

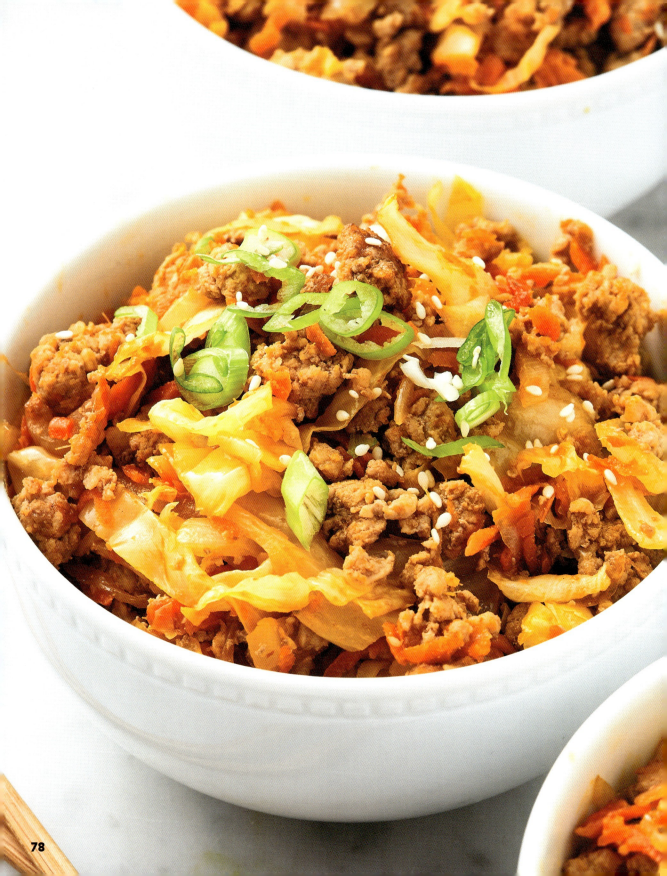

EGG ROLL BOWLS

TOTAL TIME: 35 MIN / SERVES 4

Everyone knows the filling is the best part of an egg roll.
Now you can eat all you want in bowl form.

1 tablespoon vegetable oil

1 clove garlic, minced

1 tablespoon minced fresh ginger

1 pound ground pork

1 tablespoon sesame oil

½ onion, thinly sliced

1 cup shredded carrot

¼ green cabbage, thinly sliced

¼ cup soy sauce

1 tablespoon sriracha

1 green onion, thinly sliced

1 tablespoon sesame seeds, for garnish

1 In a large skillet over medium heat, heat vegetable oil. Add garlic and ginger and cook until fragrant, 1 to 2 minutes. Add pork and cook until no pink remains.

2 Push pork to the side and add sesame oil. Add onion, shredded carrots, and cabbage. Stir to combine with meat and add soy sauce and sriracha. Cook until cabbage is tender, 5 to 8 minutes.

3 Transfer mixture to serving dish and garnish with green onions and sesame seeds before serving.

Nutrition (per serving): 420 calories, 22 g protein, 11 g carbohydrates, 3 g fiber, 5 g sugar, 32 g fat, 10 g saturated fat, 710 mg sodium

BACON-WRAPPED MEATLOAF

TOTAL TIME: 1 HR 15 MIN / SERVES 6

This meatloaf is topped with bacon slices, lending an insane amount of flavor. Almond flour acts as a binder, while soy sauce packs a punch of umami.

Cooking spray
1 tablespoon extra-virgin olive oil
1 medium onion, chopped
1 stalk celery, chopped
3 cloves garlic, minced
1 teaspoon dried oregano
1 teaspoon chili powder
2 pounds ground beef
1 cup shredded cheddar
½ cup almond flour
¼ cup grated Parmesan
2 large eggs
1 tablespoon low-sodium soy sauce
Kosher salt
Freshly ground black pepper
6 thin strips bacon

1. Preheat oven to 400°. Grease a medium baking dish with cooking spray. In a medium skillet over medium heat, heat oil. Add onion and celery and cook until soft, 5 minutes. Stir in garlic, oregano, and chili powder and cook until fragrant, 1 minute. Let mixture cool slightly.

2. In a large bowl, combine ground beef, vegetable mixture, cheddar, almond flour, Parmesan, eggs, and soy sauce, and season with salt and pepper. Shape into a large loaf in baking dish, then lay bacon slices on top.

3. Bake until bacon is crispy and beef is cooked through, about 1 hour. If bacon is cooking too quickly, cover dish with foil.

Nutrition (per serving): 450 calories, 46 g protein, 6 g carbohydrates, 2 g fiber, 1 g sugar, 27 g fat, 10 g saturated fat, 530 mg sodium

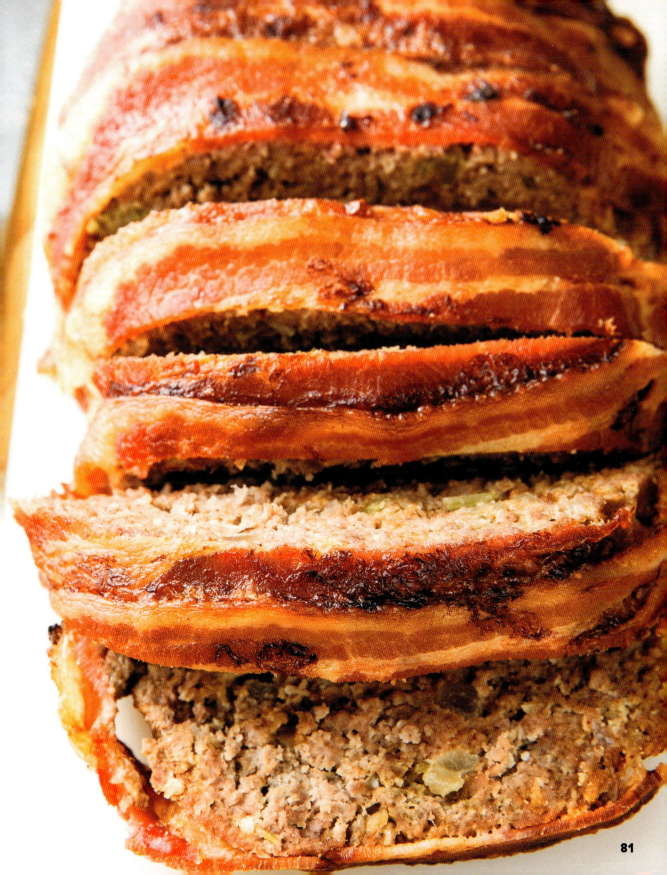

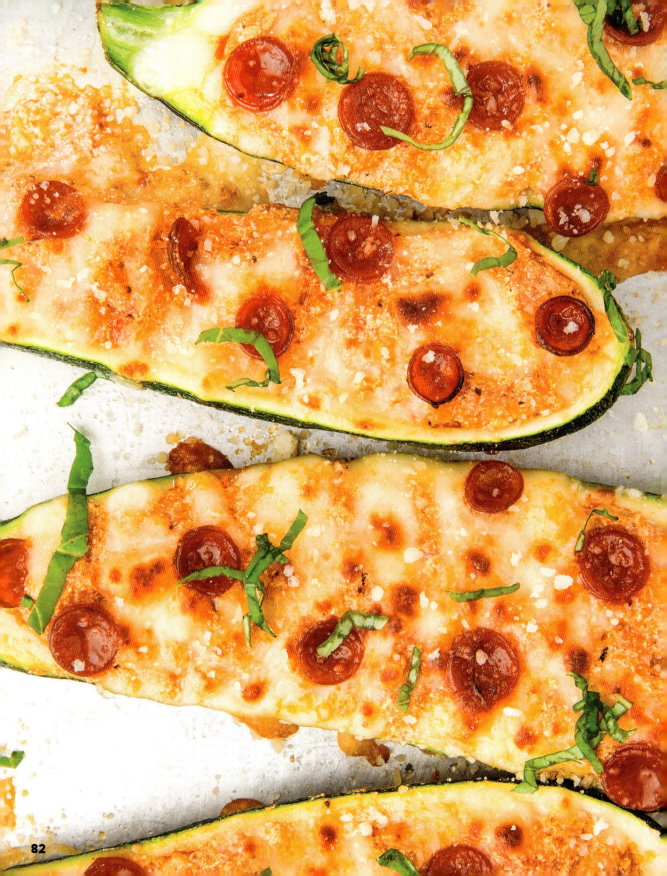

PIZZA-STUFFED ZUCCHINI

TOTAL TIME: 40 MIN / SERVES 4

Eating your veggies isn't so hard. Especially when your veggies are stuffed with melty cheese, marinara sauce, and mini pepperonis.

4 medium zucchinis
1 small onion
1 tablespoon olive oil
Kosher salt
Freshly ground black pepper
¾ cup marinara sauce
1 cup ricotta cheese
1¼ cups shredded mozzarella, divided
¼ cup grated Parmesan, plus more for garnish
1 teaspoon Italian seasoning
⅓ cup mini pepperoni slices or quartered regular pepperoni
Chopped basil, for garnish

1. Preheat oven to 450°. Halve each zucchini lengthwise. Using a spoon, remove flesh from the zucchini. Place zucchini shells in a large baking dish.

2. Meanwhile, finely chop zucchini flesh. Using a box grater, grate the onion. Heat oil in a medium nonstick skillet over medium-high heat. Add onions and chopped zucchini, cooking until soft, 6 to 8 minutes. Transfer mixture to a medium bowl and add salt, pepper, marinara sauce, ricotta, ¾ cup mozzarella cheese, Parmesan, and Italian seasoning. Stir well to combine.

3. Divide mixture among zucchini shells. Sprinkle with remaining ½ cup mozzarella. Top with pepperoni slices. Bake until golden brown, 20 to 30 minutes.

4. Garnish with Parmesan and basil before serving.

Nutrition (per serving): 330 calories, 21 g protein, 10 g carbohydrates, 1 g fiber, 1 g sugar, 23 g fat, 11 g saturated fat, 810 mg sodium

BISCUITS & GRAVY

TOTAL TIME: 30 MIN / SERVES 6

These cheddary biscuits are EVERYTHING. Slather them with our sausage gravy or use them to make a bomb avocado toast.

FOR THE BISCUITS:
Cooking spray
1 cup almond flour
2 large eggs beaten
½ cup shredded cheddar
½ cup sour cream
1 tablespoon baking powder
½ teaspoon garlic powder
¼ teaspoon kosher salt

FOR THE GRAVY:
1 pound ground breakfast sausage
2 tablespoons almond flour
¼ cup low-sodium chicken broth
¾ cup heavy cream
Freshly ground black pepper

1. Preheat the oven to 425° and grease a muffin tin with cooking spray. In a medium bowl, stir almond flour, eggs, cheddar cheese, sour cream, baking powder, garlic powder, and salt until combined.

2. Divide biscuit dough among 6 muffin cups. Bake until golden and cooked through, 12 to 14 minutes. Let cool slightly.

3. Meanwhile, in a large skillet over medium-high heat, cook sausage, breaking up meat with a wooden spoon, until seared and no longer pink, 8 to 10 minutes. Stir in almond flour and let cook 1 minute. Stirring constantly, add chicken broth and cream, and cook until thickened, about 5 minutes. Season with pepper.

4. Run a butter knife around edge of each muffin tin cup to loosen and remove biscuits. Split each biscuit in half and spoon gravy over each side.

Nutrition (per serving): 500 calories, 27 g protein, 7 g carbohydrates, 2 g fiber, 2 g sugar, 42 g fat, 17 g saturated fat, 940 mg sodium

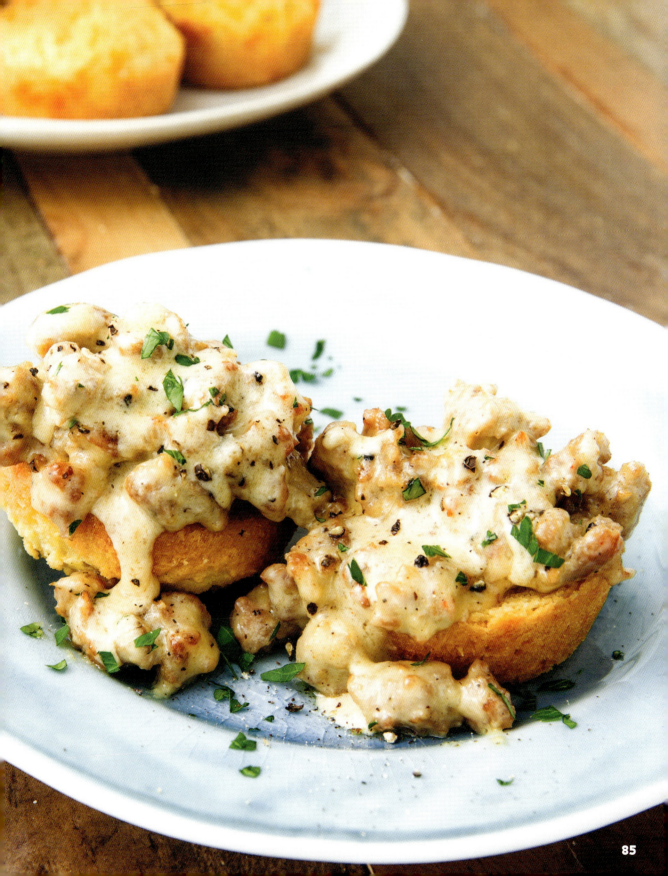

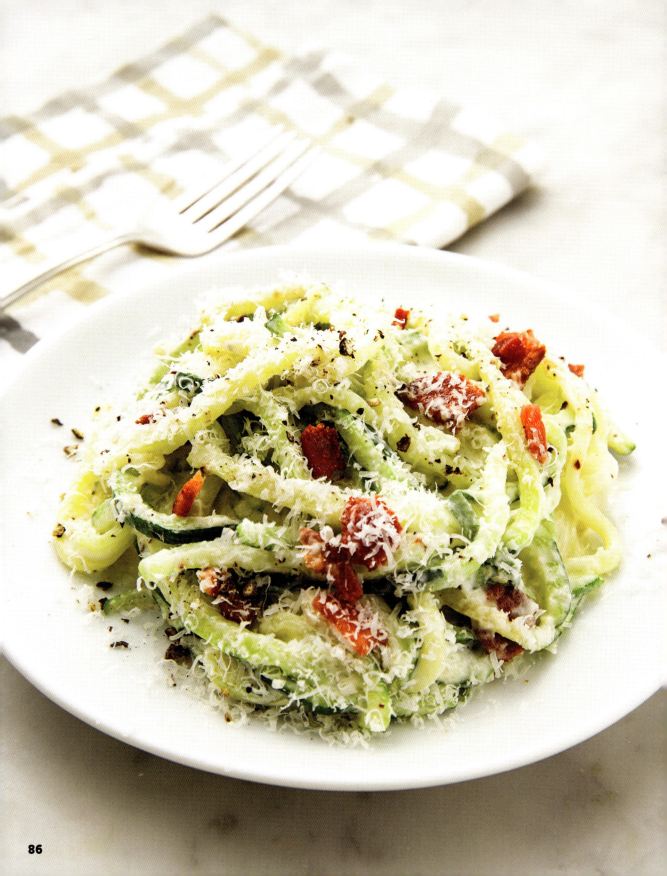

ZOODLE ALFREDO WITH BACON

TOTAL TIME: 20 MIN / SERVES 4

This decadent, luxurious sauce is rich with cream and bacon. Better yet, the zucchini noodles are great at soaking up the sauce.

½ pound bacon, chopped
1 shallot, chopped
2 cloves garlic, minced
¼ cup white wine
1½ cups heavy cream
½ cup grated Parmesan cheese, plus more for garnish
1 (16-ounce) container zucchini noodles
Freshly ground black pepper

1. In a large skillet over medium heat, cook bacon until crispy, 8 minutes. Drain on a paper towel–lined plate.

2. Pour off all but 2 tablespoons of bacon grease, then add shallots. Cook until soft, about 2 minutes, then add the garlic and cook until fragrant, about 30 seconds. Add wine and cook until reduced by half.

3. Add heavy cream and bring mixture to a boil. Reduce heat to low and stir in Parmesan. Cook until sauce has thickened slightly, about 2 minutes. Add zucchini noodles and toss until completely coated in sauce. Remove from heat and stir in cooked bacon.

4. Garnish with black pepper and more Parmesan before serving.

Nutrition (per serving): 500 calories, 14 g protein, 9 g carbohydrates, 1 g fiber, 4 g sugar, 44 g fat, 25 g saturated fat, 520 mg sodium

GARLIC ROSEMARY PORK CHOPS

TOTAL TIME: 30 MIN / SERVES 4

Garlic butter makes everything better, especially these pork chops.

4 pork loin chops

Kosher salt

Freshly ground black pepper

½ cup (1 stick) butter, melted

1 tablespoon freshly minced rosemary

2 cloves garlic, minced

1 tablespoon extra-virgin olive oil

1. Preheat oven to 375°. Season pork chops with salt and pepper.

2. In a small bowl mix together butter, rosemary, and garlic. Set aside.

3. In an oven-safe skillet over medium heat, heat olive oil then add pork chops. Sear until golden, 4 minutes, flip and cook 4 minutes more. Brush pork chops generously with garlic butter.

4. Place skillet in oven and bake until cooked through, 10 to 12 minutes. Serve with more garlic butter.

Nutrition (per serving): 460 calories, 39 g protein, 1 g carbohydrates, 0 g fiber, 0 g sugar, 33 g fat, 17 g saturated fat, 310 mg sodium

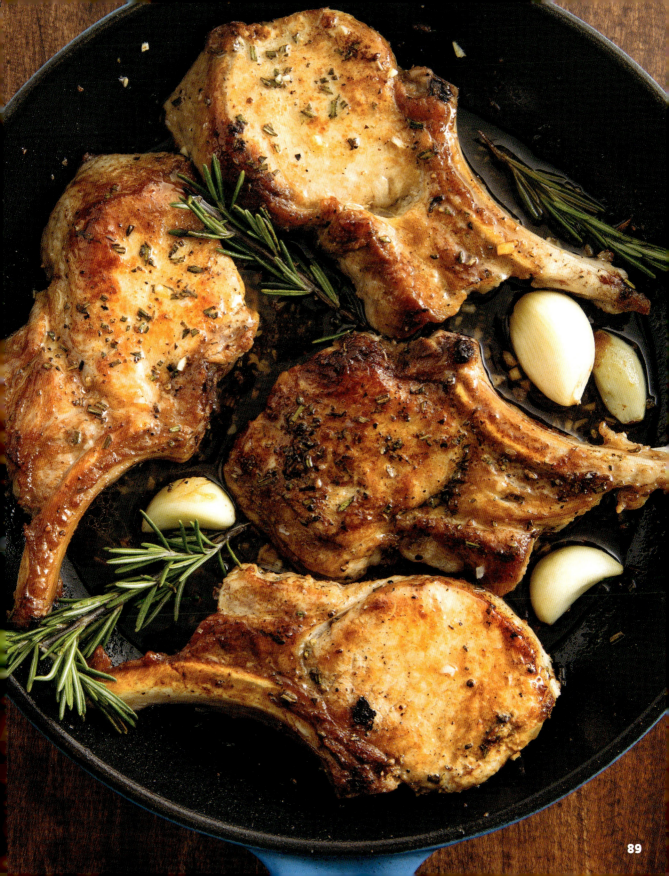

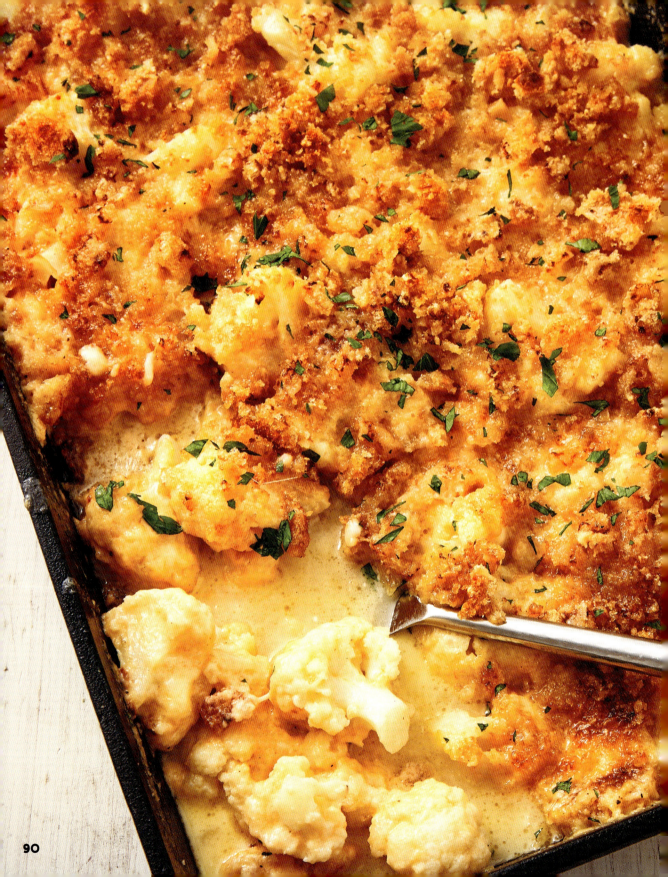

MAC & CHEESE

TOTAL TIME: 1 HR 20 MIN / SERVES 8

If you're keto, you know there are a lot of no-nos in classic mac & cheese. This version takes out all the trouble children (ahem, PASTA) *without* sacrificing flavor.

FOR THE MAC & CHEESE:
- Butter, for baking dish
- 2 medium heads cauliflower, cut into florets
- 2 tablespoons extra-virgin olive oil
- Kosher salt
- 1 cup heavy cream
- 6 ounces cream cheese, cut into cubes
- 4 cups shredded cheddar
- 2 cups shredded mozzarella
- 1 tablespoon hot sauce (optional)
- Freshly ground black pepper

FOR THE TOPPING:
- 4 ounces pork rinds, crushed
- ¼ cup freshly grated Parmesan
- 1 tablespoon extra-virgin olive oil
- 2 tablespoons freshly chopped parsley, for garnish

1. Preheat the oven to 375° and butter a 13"-x-9" baking dish. In a large bowl, toss cauliflower with oil and season with salt. Spread cauliflower onto 2 large baking sheets and roast until tender and lightly golden, about 40 minutes.

2. Meanwhile, in a large pot over medium heat, heat cream. Bring up to a simmer, then decrease heat to low and stir in cheeses until melted. Remove from heat, add hot sauce if using and season with salt and pepper, then fold in roasted cauliflower. Taste and season more if needed.

3. Transfer mixture to prepared baking dish. In a medium bowl stir to combine pork rinds, Parmesan, and oil. Sprinkle mixture in an even layer over cauliflower and cheese.

4. Bake until golden, 15 minutes. If desired, turn oven to broil to toast topping further, about 2 minutes.

5. Garnish with parsley before serving.

Nutrition (per serving): 669 calories, 34 g protein, 12 g carbohydrates, 3 g fiber, 5 g sugar, 55 g fat, 29 g saturated fat, 1,214 mg sodium

CAULIFLOWER BAKED ZITI

TOTAL TIME: 1 HR 10 MIN / SERVES 6

Ok fine. There's not actually any ziti in this recipe. Honestly though, you won't even notice. The blanched cauliflower does a great job replacing the pasta — just make sure to drain it well before tossing it with the sauce.

1 tablespoon extra-virgin olive oil

1 medium onion, chopped

2 garlic cloves, minced

Pinch red pepper flakes

1 pound ground beef

Kosher salt

Freshly ground black pepper

2 tablespoons tomato paste

1 teaspoon dried oregano

1 (28-ounce) can crushed tomatoes

2 tablespoons thinly sliced basil, plus more for garnish

1 large head of cauliflower, (about 3 cups) cut into florets, blanched, and drained well

1½ cups fresh ricotta

2 cups shredded mozzarella

½ cup freshly grated Parmesan

1. Preheat oven to 375°. In a large saucepan over medium heat, heat oil. Add onion and cook, stirring often, until onion is soft, about 5 minutes. Stir in garlic and red pepper flakes and cook for one minute. Add meat and season with salt and pepper. Cook until no longer pink, 6 minutes. Drain fat.

2. Return saucepan over medium heat and add tomato paste and oregano. Cook for 2 minutes more, until slightly darkened. Add crushed tomatoes and bring sauce to a simmer, reduce heat and cook, stirring occasionally, until slightly reduced and flavors have melded, 10 to 15 minutes. Remove from heat and stir in basil.

3. In a large bowl, pour sauce over cauliflower and stir to combine. In a large baking dish, place half the cauliflower in an even layer. Dollop all over with half the ricotta, and sprinkle with half the mozzarella and Parmesan. Add the rest of the cauliflower in an even layer on top, and top with remaining cheeses.

4. Bake until cheese is melty and golden, 25 minutes. Garnish with basil before serving.

Nutrition (per serving): 467 calories, 35 g protein, 19 carbohydrates, 4 g fiber, 9 g sugar, 29 g fat, 14 g saturated fat, 877 mg sodium

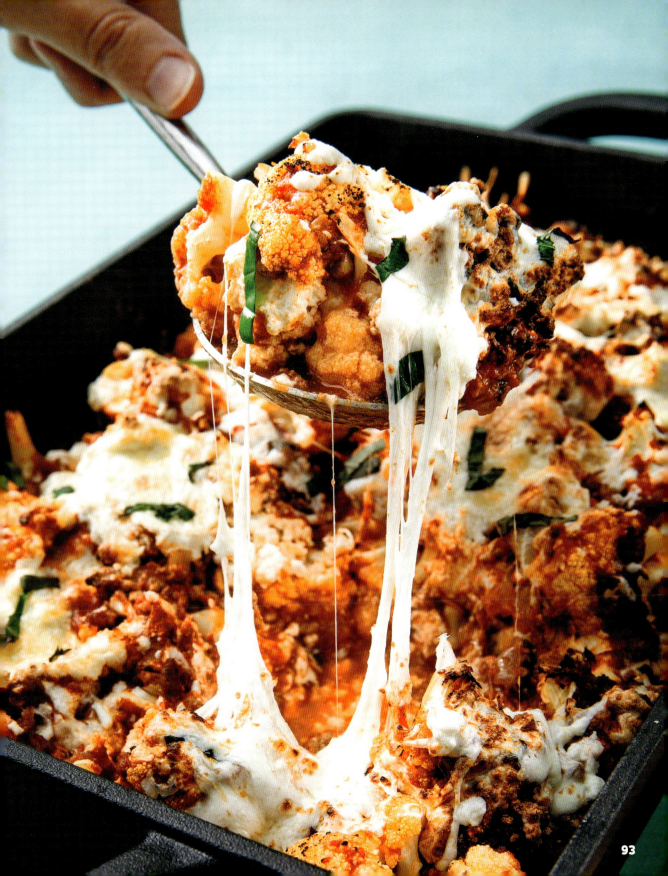

CHICKEN PICCATA

TOTAL TIME: 30 MIN / SERVES 4

This one-pan lemony chicken comes together in just 30 minutes.

1 tablespoon extra-virgin olive oil

4 bone-in, skin-on chicken thighs

Kosher salt

Freshly ground black pepper

2 tablespoons butter

3 cloves garlic, minced

¼ cup dry white wine

Juice of 1 lemon

2 tablespoons capers

1 lemon, sliced

Freshly chopped parsley, for garnish

1. In a large ovenproof skillet over medium-high heat, heat oil. Season chicken with salt and pepper and cook until golden and no longer pink, 8 minutes per side. Transfer to a plate. Discard half the chicken juice from skillet and reduce heat to low.

2. To skillet, add butter, garlic, wine, lemon juice, and capers and bring to a simmer. Add lemon slices and return chicken thighs to skillet. Let chicken simmer in sauce 5 minutes, then garnish with parsley before serving.

Nutrition (per serving): 180 calories, 14 g protein, 1 g carbohydrates, 0 g fiber, 0 g sugar, 12 g fat, 5 g saturated fat, 230 mg sodium

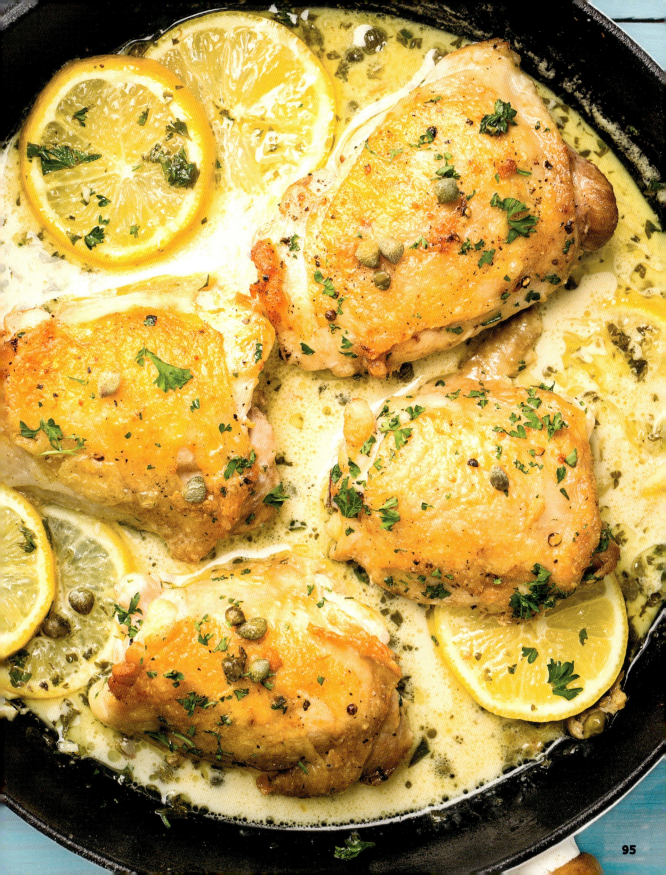

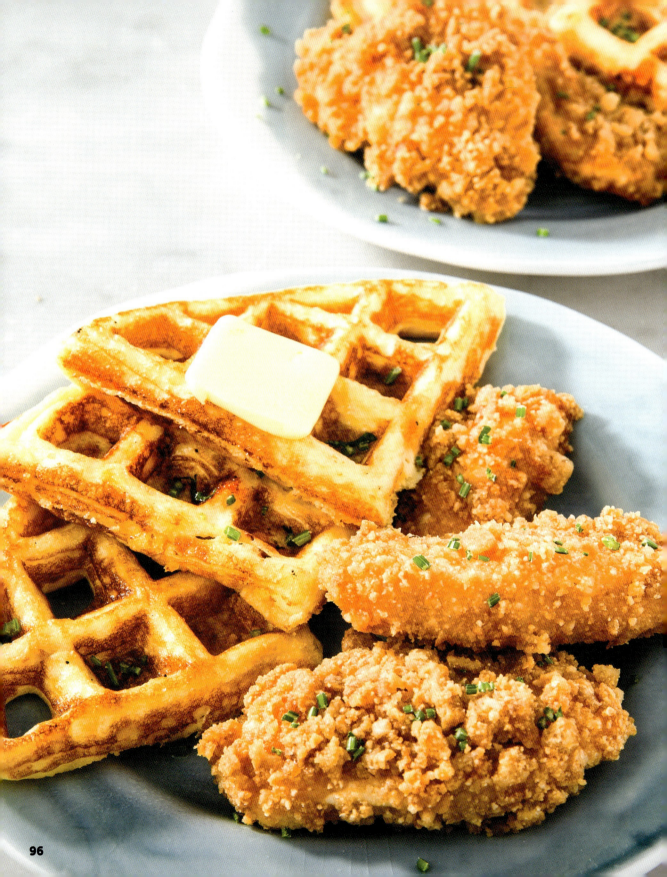

CRISPY CHICKEN & WAFFLES

TOTAL TIME: 1 HR 5 MIN / SERVES 6

Crunchy pork rind coated chicken tenders top gluten-free waffles for an indulgent breakfast you can feel good about.

FOR THE CHICKEN:
- Cooking spray
- 4 ounces pork rinds
- 1 cup freshly grated Parmesan
- 1 large egg
- 2 tablespoons mayonnaise
- 2 tablespoons water
- Kosher salt
- Freshly ground black pepper
- 1 pound boneless skinless chicken breasts, cut into strips

FOR THE WAFFLES:
- 4 large eggs
- 2 cups almond flour
- 1 cup shredded cheddar
- 1 cup milk
- 1 cup sour cream
- 1 teaspoon baking powder
- Kosher salt
- Freshly ground black pepper
- Cooking spray
- 2 tablespoons freshly chopped chives, for garnish
- Butter (optional)

1. Preheat the oven to 425°. Line a baking sheet with parchment paper and grease generously with cooking spray. Add pork rinds to a food processor and pulse until fine crumbs form. Transfer to a shallow dish and combine with Parmesan.

2. In a medium bowl, whisk together egg, mayo, and water. Season with salt and pepper.

3. Dip chicken pieces in egg mixture, letting excess liquid drip off. Coat chicken in pork-rind mixture, pressing to adhere, and place on baking sheet.

4. Bake until golden, 25 to 30 minutes.

5. Meanwhile, make the waffles: Preheat a waffle iron. In a large bowl, whisk eggs, then whisk in almond flour, cheddar, milk, sour cream, and baking powder and season with salt and pepper. Grease waffle iron with cooking spray. Following waffle maker directions, add ½ cup batter and cook until golden, 4 to 5 minutes. Repeat with remaining batter.

6. Serve chicken tenders with waffles and garnish with chives and butter.

Nutrition (per serving): 720 calories, 50 g protein, 14 g carbohydrates, 4 g fiber, 5 g sugar, 52 g fat, 16 g saturated fat, 1,119 mg sodium

JALAPEÑO POPPER CHICKEN CASSEROLE

TOTAL TIME: 45 MIN / SERVES 6

If you have to order jalapeño poppers whenever you see them on the menu, this low-carb chicken casserole is about to become your favorite weeknight dinner.

Cooking spray

1½ tablespoons extra-virgin olive oil, divided

2 pounds boneless, skinless chicken breasts, sliced into strips

Kosher salt

Freshly ground black pepper

1 red bell pepper, chopped

3 to 4 jalapeños, chopped

1 (8-ounce) package cream cheese, cubed

¼ cup mayonnaise

1 cup shredded cheddar, divided

4 slices bacon, chopped, for garnish

1. Preheat oven to 400° and grease an 8"-x-8" baking dish with cooking spray. In a large skillet over medium-high heat, heat 1 tablespoon oil. Season chicken with salt and pepper then cook until seared and no longer pink in middle, about 6 minutes per side. Remove from heat and let cool slightly before chopping into bite-size pieces.

2. In the same skillet over medium heat, heat remaining ½ tablespoon oil and cook bell pepper and jalapeños until soft, about 5 minutes. Add cream cheese, mayo, and chopped chicken, stirring until cream cheese melts. Stir in ¾ cup cheddar and remove from heat.

3. Add chicken mixture to prepared baking dish and top with remaining ¼ cup cheddar. Bake until cheese is melty and bubbly, 15 to 20 minutes.

4. Meanwhile, in a medium skillet over medium heat, cook bacon until crispy, about 8 minutes. Drain on a paper towel-lined plate.

5. Garnish casserole with cooked bacon pieces before serving.

Nutrition (per serving): 440 calories, 43 g protein, 5 g carbohydrates, 0 g fiber, 2 g sugar, 29 g fat, 13 g saturated fat, 460 mg sodium

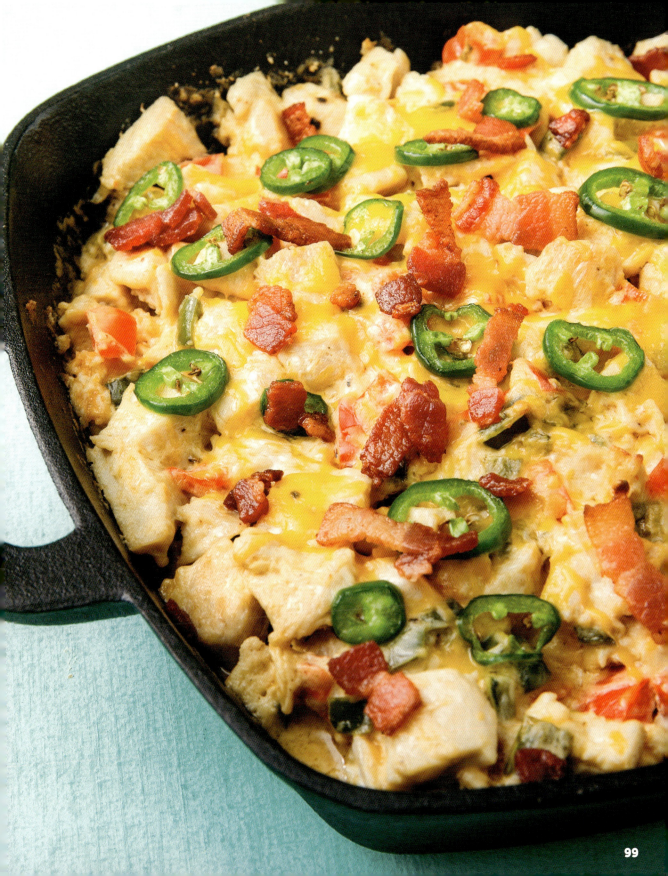

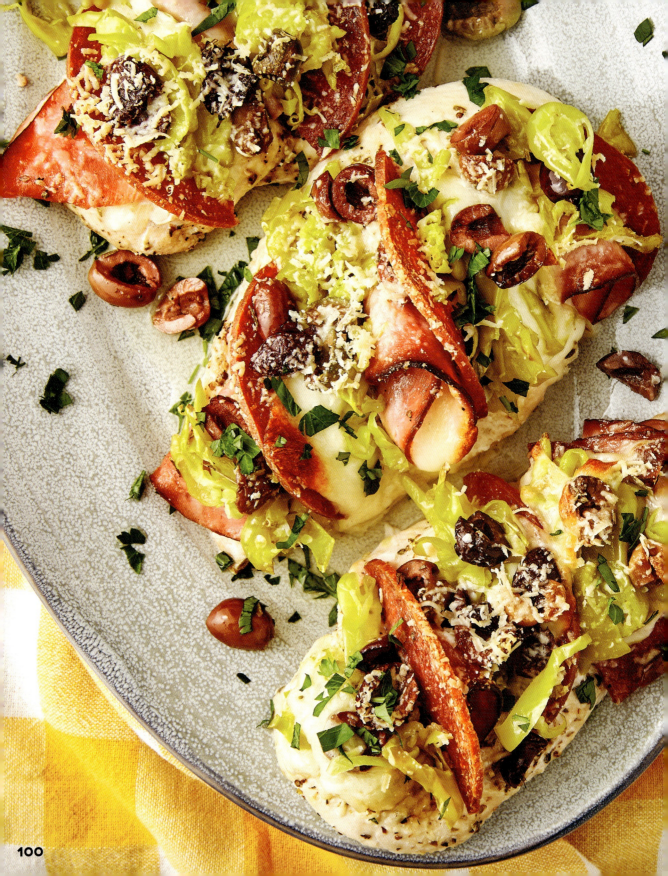

ANTIPASTO STUFFED CHICKEN

TOTAL TIME: 40 MIN / SERVES 4

We love this technique for stuffing chicken. When loaded with vegetables, meat, and cheese, it turns a chicken breast into a full-blown meal.

4 boneless, skinless chicken breasts

2 tablespoons extra-virgin olive oil

1 teaspoon dried oregano

½ teaspoon garlic powder

Kosher salt

Freshly ground black pepper

¼ pound deli ham

¼ pound pepperoni slices

4 slices provolone, halved

1 cup drained and sliced pepperoncini

⅓ cup chopped assorted olives

¼ cup grated Parmesan

Freshly chopped parsley for garnish

1. Preheat oven to 400°. Place chicken on a cutting board and make 5 slits in each breast, being careful not to cut through completely. Transfer to a small baking sheet.

2. Drizzle oil over chicken and season with oregano, garlic powder, salt and pepper.

3. Stuff each chicken breast with ham, pepperoni, provolone, and pepperoncini, then sprinkle with olives and Parmesan.

4. Bake until chicken is cooked through and no longer pink, about 25 minutes. Garnish with parsley before serving.

Nutrition (per serving): 560 calories, 45 g protein, 6 g carbohydrates, 0 g fiber, 0 g sugar, 40 g fat, 13 g saturated fat, 1880 mg sodium

CREAMY TUSCAN CHICKEN

TOTAL TIME: 40 MIN / SERVES 4

The garlicky cream sauce on this chicken recipe is stupid good. Eat it over mashed cauliflower so you can soak up every drop.

1 tablespoon extra-virgin olive oil

4 boneless, skinless chicken breasts

Kosher salt

Freshly ground black pepper

1 teaspoon dried oregano

3 tablespoons unsalted butter

3 cloves garlic, minced

1½ cups cherry tomatoes

2 cups baby spinach

½ cup heavy cream

¼ cup freshly grated Parmesan

Lemon wedges, for serving

1. In a skillet over medium heat, heat oil. Add chicken and season with salt, pepper, and oregano. Cook until golden and no longer pink, 8 minutes per side. Remove from skillet and set aside.

2. In the same skillet over medium heat, melt butter. Stir in garlic and cook until fragrant, about 1 minute. Add cherry tomatoes and season with salt and pepper. Cook until tomatoes are beginning to burst then add spinach and cook until spinach is beginning to wilt.

3. Stir in heavy cream and Parmesan and bring mixture to a simmer. Reduce heat to low and simmer until sauce is slightly reduced, about 3 minutes. Return chicken to skillet and cook until heated through, 5 to 7 minutes. Remove from heat, squeeze with lemon and serve.

Nutrition (per serving): 380 calories, 29 g protein, 5 g carbohydrates, 1 g fiber, 2 g sugar, 28 g fat, 14 g saturated fat, 250 mg sodium

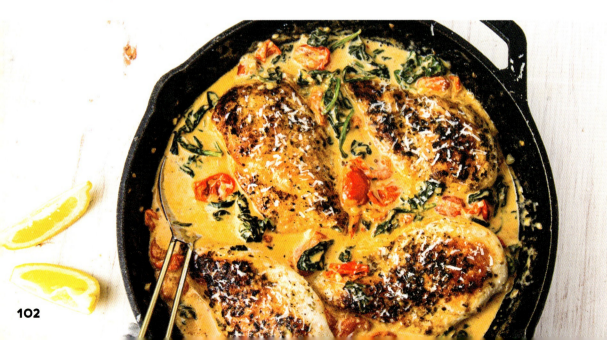

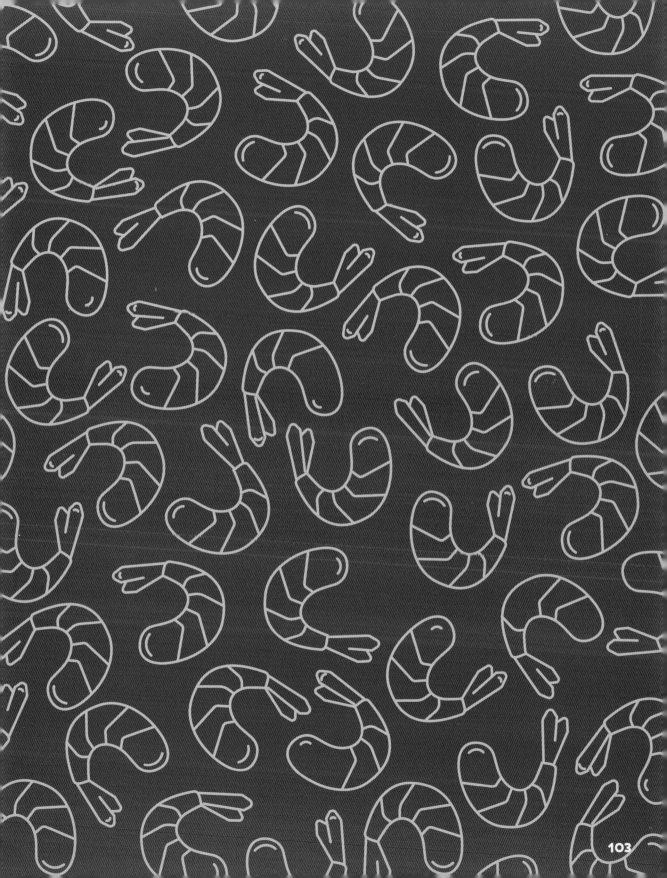

INSANELY EASY SEAFOOD & VEGGIES

Chilean Sea Bass with Spinach-Avocado Pesto	105
Best Greek Salad	106
Tuscan Butter Salmon	109
Avocado Crab Boats	110
Breaded Shrimp	111
Rosemary-Dijon Salmon	112
Bruschetta Swordfish	115
Grilled Salmon & Lemony Asparagus Foil Packs	116
Spinach-Artichoke Stuffed Mushrooms	118
Creamed Spinach Stuffed Salmon	119
Garlicky Lemon Mahi-Mahi	121
Lemon Butter Baked Tilapia	122
Garlicky Shrimp Zucchini Pasta	124
Pesto Shrimp Skewers with Cauliflower Mash	125
Perfect Baked Cod	126
Zucchini Ravioli	129
Caprese Stuffed Avocados	130

CHILEAN SEA BASS WITH SPINACH-AVOCADO PESTO

TOTAL TIME: 30 MIN / SERVES 4

Revamp your classic pesto recipe with avocado, which makes it super creamy and packs in the healthy fats you need.

4 pieces (about 2 pounds) wild Chilean sea bass

Kosher salt

Freshly ground black pepper

2 cups baby spinach

½ cup fresh parsley, chopped, plus more for garnish

1 clove of garlic, smashed

¼ cup walnuts, chopped

2 teaspoons fresh lemon juice

Extra virgin olive oil

1 avocado, pitted and peeled

1 pound asparagus, ends trimmed

2 lemons, cut in half

Flaky sea salt

1. Season sea bass with salt and pepper; set aside.

2. In the bowl of a food processor, add spinach, parsley, garlic, walnuts, lemon juice, ¼ cup olive oil, ½ teaspoon Kosher salt and ¼ tsp pepper. Pulse 2 to 3 times. Add avocado and pulse until well blended but the pesto sauce still maintains some texture.

3. Preheat a large cast-iron skillet over high heat. Heat 1 tablespoon olive oil until very hot and almost smoking. Sear sea bass on each side for 3 minutes. Transfer to a plate and let it rest for a minute.

4. Meanwhile, return cast-iron skillet to medium-high heat. Add 1 tsp olive oil, asparagus, and ½ tsp salt. Sauté for 5 minutes, transfer to a plate for serving. Place lemons cut side down in the skillet, turn heat to high and sear lemon for 1 minute.

5. Serve sea bass on bed of asparagus and top with pesto and seared lemon. Garnish with parsley and a sprinkle of sea salt.

Nutrition (per serving): 410 calories, 58 g protein, 10 g carbohydrates, 6 g fiber, 2 g sugar, 15 g fat, 2.5 g saturated fat, 230 mg sodium

BEST GREEK SALAD

TOTAL TIME: 15 MIN / SERVES 4

A classic we turn to again and again. You'll want to use the lemony dressing on everything.

FOR THE SALAD:

1 pint grape or cherry tomatoes, halved

1 cucumber, thinly sliced into half moons

1 cup halved Kalamata olives

½ red onion, thinly sliced

¾ cup crumbled feta

Parsley, for garnish

FOR THE DRESSING:

2 tablespoons red wine vinegar

Juice of ½ lemon

1 teaspoon dried oregano

Kosher salt

Freshly ground black pepper

¼ cup extra-virgin olive oil

1 In a large bowl, stir together tomatoes, cucumber, olives, and onion. Gently fold in feta.

2 In a small bowl, make dressing: Combine vinegar, lemon juice, and oregano and season with salt and pepper. Slowly add olive oil, whisking to combine.

3 Drizzle dressing over salad and garnish with parsley.

Nutrition (per serving): 230 calories, 5 g protein, 7 g carbohydrates, 2 g fiber, 4 g sugar, 20 g fat, 6 g saturated fat, 320 mg sodium

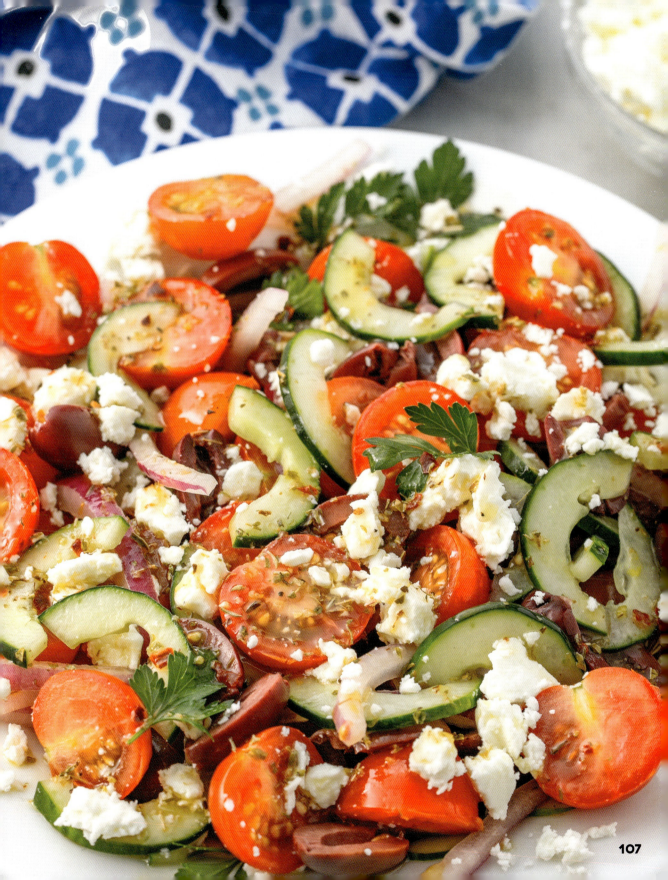

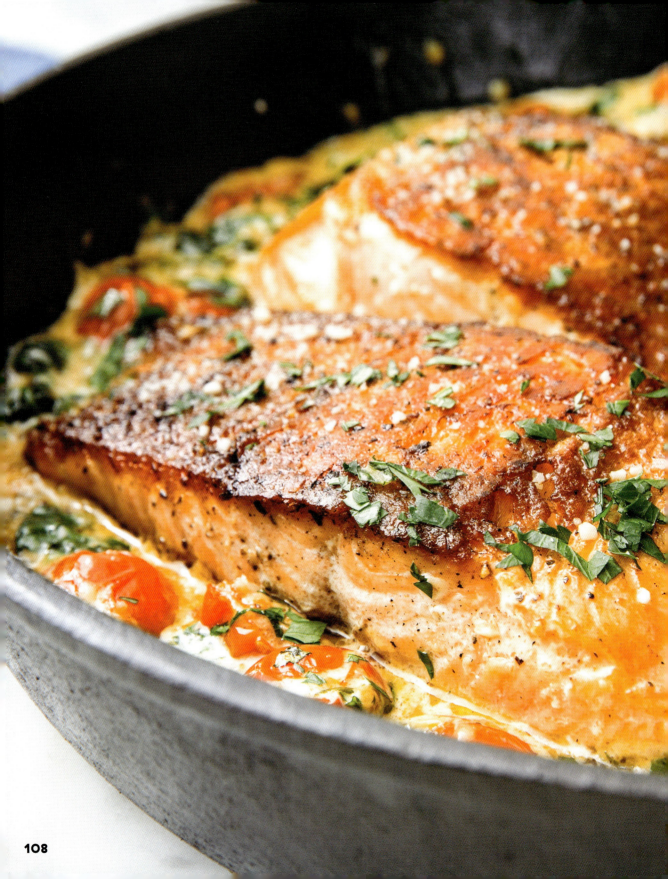

TUSCAN BUTTER SALMON

TOTAL TIME: 45 MIN / SERVES 4

There's a reason this is one of our most popular recipes of all time. The tomato-and-basil cream sauce with Parmesan is unbelievably dreamy.

2 tablespoons extra-virgin olive oil

4 (6-ounce) salmon fillets, patted dry with paper towels

Kosher salt

Freshly ground black pepper

3 tablespoons butter

3 cloves garlic, minced

1½ cups halved cherry tomatoes

2 cups baby spinach

½ cup heavy cream

¼ cup freshly grated Parmesan

¼ cup chopped herbs (such as basil and parsley), plus more for garnish

Lemon wedges, for serving (optional)

1. In a large skillet over medium-high heat, heat oil. Season salmon all over with salt and pepper. When oil is shimmering but not smoking, add salmon skin side up and cook until deeply golden, about 6 minutes. Flip over and cook 2 minutes more. Transfer to a plate.

2. Reduce heat to medium and add butter. When butter has melted, stir in garlic and cook until fragrant, about 1 minute. Add cherry tomatoes and season with salt and pepper. Cook until tomatoes are beginning to burst, then add spinach. Cook until spinach is beginning to wilt.

3. Stir in heavy cream, Parmesan, and herbs and bring mixture to a simmer. Reduce heat to low and simmer until sauce is slightly reduced, about 3 minutes.

4. Return salmon back to skillet and spoon over sauce. Simmer until salmon is cooked through, about 3 minutes more.

5. Garnish with more herbs and squeeze lemon on top before serving.

Nutrition (per serving): 531 calories, 40 g protein, 6 g carbohydrates, 1 g fiber, 2 g sugar, 38 g fat, 16 g saturated fat, 505 mg sodium

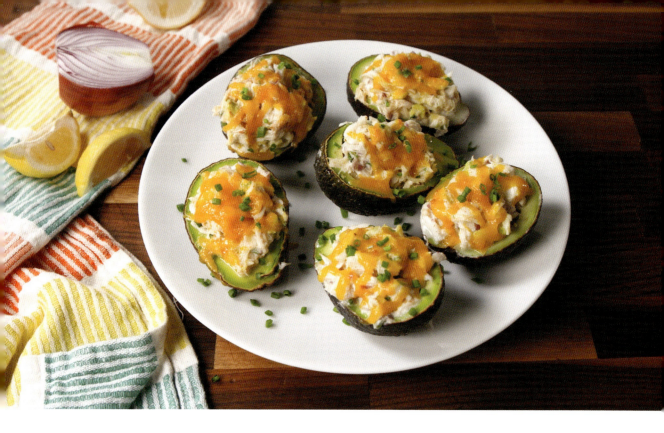

AVOCADO CRAB BOATS

TOTAL TIME: 10 MIN / SERVES 4

What *can't* avocados do? These boats are filled with creamy, cheesy crab meat. Not a crab fan? You can sub in canned tuna or cooked and chopped shrimp.

12 ounces lump crab meat
⅓ cup Greek yogurt
½ red onion, minced
2 tablespoons chopped chives
3 tablespoons lemon juice
½ teaspoon cayenne pepper
Kosher salt
2 avocados, halved and pitted
1 cup shredded cheddar

1 In a medium bowl, stir together crab meat, yogurt, onion, chives, lemon juice, and cayenne, and season with salt.

2 Scoop out avocados to create bowls, leaving a small border. Dice scooped-out avocado and fold into crab mixture.

3 Preheat broiler. Fill avocado bowls with crab mixture and top with cheddar. Broil until cheese is just melted, about 1 minute. Serve immediately.

Nutrition (per serving): 350 calories, 30 g protein, 9 g carbohydrates, 5 g fiber, 2 g sugar, 21 g fat, 8 g saturated fat, 510 mg sodium

BREADED SHRIMP

TOTAL TIME: 35 MIN / SERVES 4

Crushed pork rinds are the secret here: They give shrimp a salty crunch every keto lover will appreciate.

FOR THE SHRIMP:

Cooking spray

6 ounces pork rinds

¼ cup grated Parmesan

1 teaspoon chili powder

½ teaspoon paprika

½ teaspoon garlic powder

½ teaspoon dried oregano

Kosher salt

Freshly ground black pepper

2 large eggs, beaten

1 pound large shrimp peeled and deveined

FOR THE SAUCE + GARNISH:

½ cup mayonnaise (or sour cream)

Juice of ½ lemon

Dash of hot sauce

Freshly chopped parsley, for garnish

1 Preheat oven to 450° and grease a large rimmed baking sheet with cooking spray. In a food processor (or in a resealable bag using a rolling pin), crush pork rinds into fine crumbs. Transfer to a medium shallow bowl and whisk in Parmesan, spices, and herbs. Season mixture with salt and pepper.

2 Pour beaten eggs into a small shallow bowl. Dredge shrimp in eggs, letting excess drip, then coat in pork rind mixture.

3 Place coated shrimp on prepared baking sheet in single layer. Bake until coating is crispy and shrimp is cooked through, 10 to 12 minutes.

4 Meanwhile, make sauce: In a small bowl, whisk together mayonnaise, lemon juice, and hot sauce. Garnish shrimp with parsley and serve with the sauce

Nutrition (per serving): 580 calories, 47 g protein, 3 g carbohydrates, 0 g fiber, 0 g sugar, 40 g fat, 10 g saturated fat, 298 mg sodium

ROSEMARY-DIJON SALMON

TOTAL TIME: 20 MIN / SERVES 4

Rubbing salmon with a mixture of grainy mustard, garlic, rosemary, and shallot takes it to the next level.

1 tablespoon grainy mustard

2 cloves garlic, finely minced

1 tablespoon shallots, finely minced

2 teaspoons fresh thyme leaves, chopped, plus more for garnish

2 teaspoons fresh rosemary, chopped

Juice of ½ lemon

Kosher salt

Freshly ground black pepper

4 (4-ounce) salmon fillets

Lemon slices, for serving

1 Heat broiler and line a baking sheet with parchment. In a small bowl, mix together mustard, garlic, shallots, thyme, rosemary, and lemon juice and season with salt and peppers. Spread mixture all over salmon fillets and broil, 7 to 8 minutes.

2 Garnish with more thyme and lemon slices before serving.

Nutrition (per serving): 570 calories, 79 g protein, 1 g carbohydrates, 0 g fiber, 0 g sugar, 26 g fat, 4 g saturated fat, 170 mg sodium

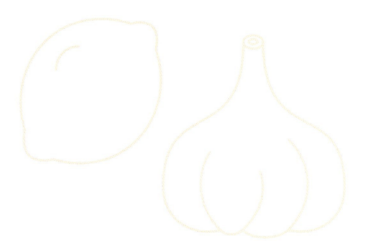

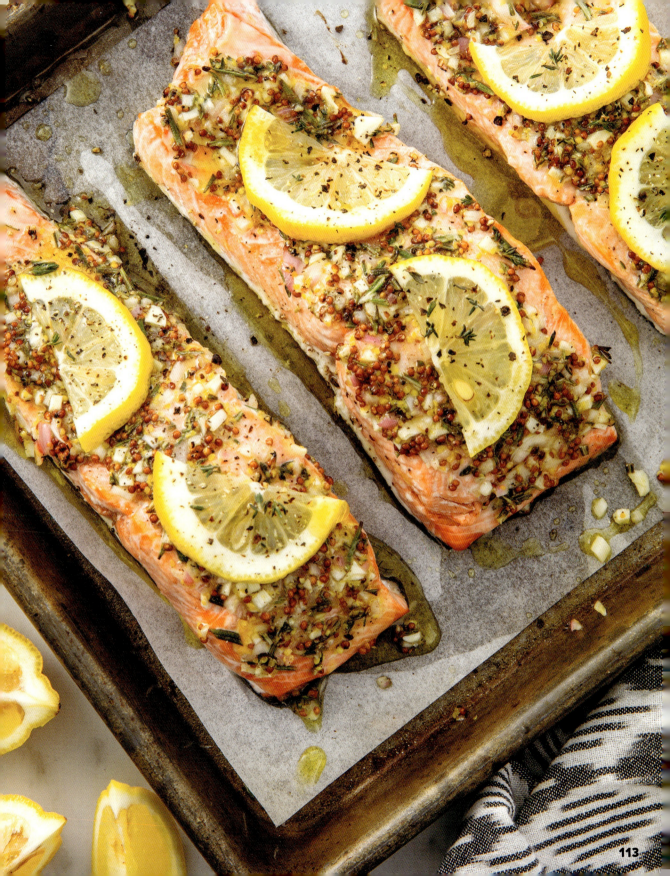

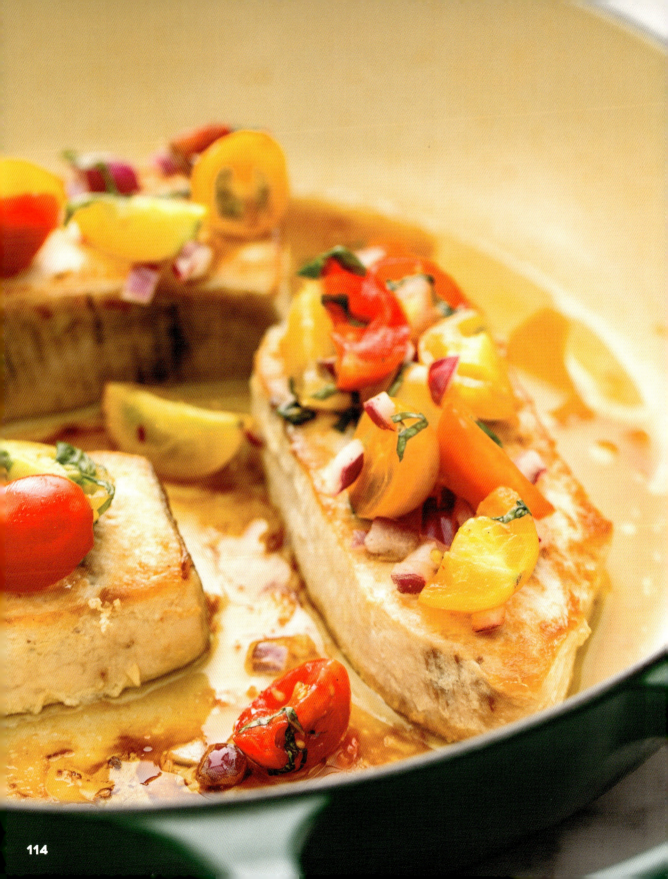

BRUSCHETTA SWORDFISH

TOTAL TIME: 20 MIN / SERVES 4

This easy tomato, onion, basil bruschetta mixture brightens up any seafood dish.

3 tablespoons extra-virgin olive oil, divided
3 swordfish steaks
Kosher salt
Freshly ground black pepper
2 pints multicolored cherry tomatoes, halved
¼ cup red onion, finely chopped
3 tablespoons thinly sliced fresh basil
Juice of ½ lemon

1. Preheat oven to 400°. In a large cast-iron skillet over high heat, heat 2 tablespoons oil. Add fish to pan and season tops with salt and pepper. Cook until fish is browned on one side, 3 to 5 minutes. Flip and season the opposite side with salt and pepper. Remove pan from heat and place into the oven.

2. Roast until swordfish is cooked through and flaky, about 10 minutes.

3. Make the fresh tomato salad: In a large bowl, combine tomatoes, onion, and basil. Add remaining tablespoon oil and the lemon juice and season with salt and pepper.

4. Spoon salad over fish before serving.

Nutrition (per serving): 270 calories, 21 g protein, 7 g carbohydrates, 2 g fiber, 4 g sugar, 18 g fat, 3 g saturated fat, 90 mg sodium

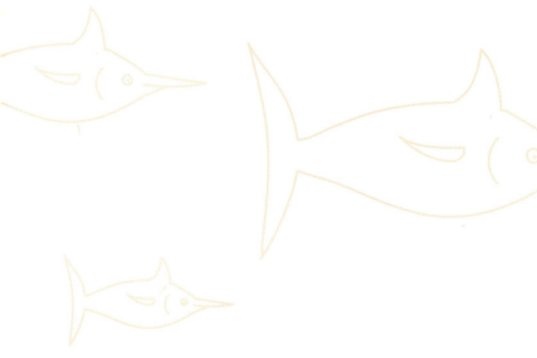

GRILLED SALMON & LEMONY ASPARAGUS FOIL PACKS

TOTAL TIME: 20 MIN / SERVES 4

These foil packs work with whatever vegetables or seafood you like. Just don't forget the dill and lemon slices.

20 asparagus spears, ends trimmed

4 (6-ounce) skin-on salmon fillets

4 tablespoons butter, divided

2 lemons, sliced

Kosher salt

Freshly ground black pepper

Torn fresh dill, for garnish

1 Lay two pieces of foil on a flat surface. Place 5 spears of asparagus on foil and top with a fillet of salmon, 1 tablespoon butter, 2 slices lemon, salt, and pepper. Loosely wrap, then repeat with remaining ingredients until you have 4 packets total.

2 Heat grill on high. Add foil packets to grill and grill until salmon is cooked through and asparagus is tender, about 10 minutes.

3 Garnish with dill before serving.

Nutrition (per serving): 360 calories, 36 g protein, 4 g carbohydrates, 2 g fiber, 2 g sugar, 22 g fat, 9 g saturated fat, 180 mg sodium

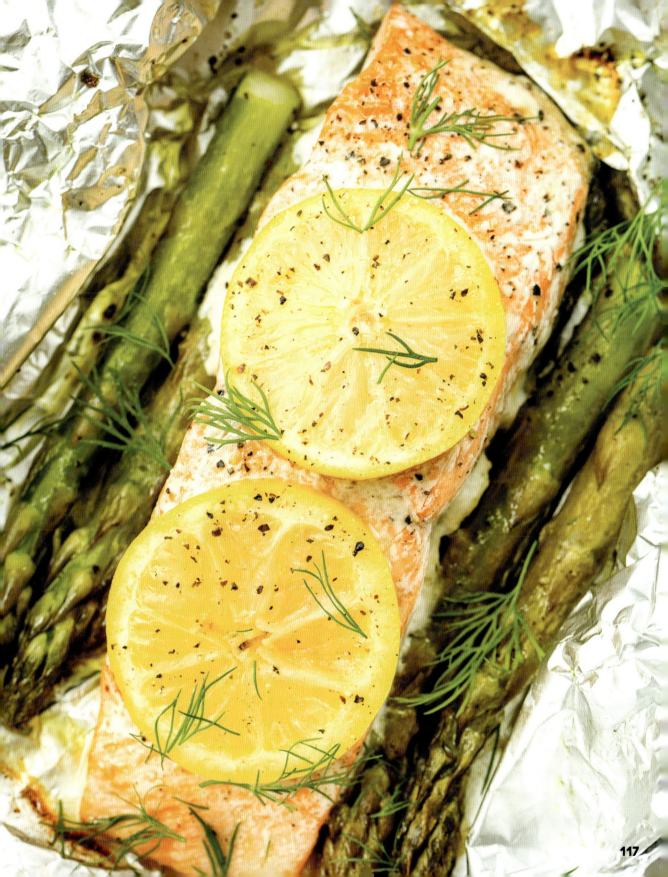

SPINACH-ARTICHOKE STUFFED MUSHROOMS

TOTAL TIME: 40 MIN / SERVES 4

If you thought traditional stuffed mushrooms were addictive, just wait until you try this twist.

4 medium portobello mushrooms, stems and gills removed

2 tablespoons extra-virgin olive oil

1 package frozen chopped spinach, thawed, drained and squeezed dry

1 (14-ounce) can artichoke hearts, drained and chopped

¼ (8-ounce) block room temperature cream cheese, cut into 20 pieces

2 tablespoons mayonnaise

2 tablespoons sour cream

1 cup shredded mozzarella, divided

½ cup grated Parmesan, divided

2 cloves garlic, minced

Red pepper flakes

Kosher salt

Freshly ground black pepper

1. Preheat oven to 375°. Brush face-down mushroom caps with olive oil. Cook on baking sheet for about 10 minutes until beginning to soften.

2. Meanwhile, combine spinach, artichoke, cream cheese, mayonnaise, sour cream, ½ cup mozzarella, ¼ cup Parmesan, garlic, and red pepper flakes in a large bowl. Season with salt and pepper to taste.

3. Flip over mushrooms and stuff each cap with an equal amount of the spinach mixture. Sprinkle tops with remaining cheeses.

4. Return pan to oven and bake for another 10 to 15 minutes, until the mushrooms are easily pierced with fork and the cheese is melted.

5. Once melted, switch oven to broil and broil the mushroom caps for a few minutes until the cheese starts to brown.

Nutrition (per serving): 470 calories, 17 g protein, 16 g carbohydrates, 5 g fiber, 5 g sugar, 39 g fat, 13 g saturated fat, 870 mg sodium

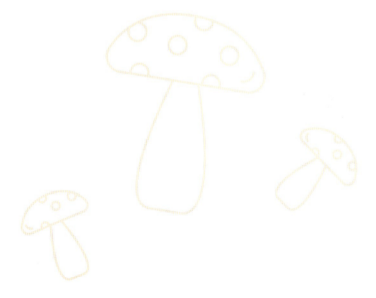

CREAMED SPINACH STUFFED SALMON

TOTAL TIME: 20 MIN / SERVES 4

Skeptical about the combination of cheese and salmon? Don't be. We promise you, it's killer.

- 4 (6-ounce) salmon fillets
- Kosher salt
- Freshly ground black pepper
- ½ (8-ounce) block cream cheese, softened
- ½ cup shredded mozzarella
- ½ cup frozen spinach, defrosted
- ¼ teaspoon garlic powder
- Pinch red pepper flakes
- 1 tablespoon extra-virgin olive oil
- 2 tablespoons butter
- Juice of ½ lemon

1. Season salmon all over with salt and pepper. In a large bowl, mix together cream cheese, mozzarella, spinach, garlic powder, and red pepper flakes.

2. Using a paring knife, slice a slit in each salmon to create a pocket. Stuff pockets with cream cheese mixture.

3. In a large skillet over medium heat, heat oil. Add salmon skin-side-down and cook until seared, about 6 minutes, then flip salmon. Add butter to skillet and squeeze lemon juice all over. Cook until skin is crispy, another 6 minutes. Serve warm.

Nutrition (per serving): 440 calories, 40 g protein, 3 g carbohydrates, 1 g fiber, 1 g sugar, 29 g fat, 12 g saturated fat, 320 mg sodium

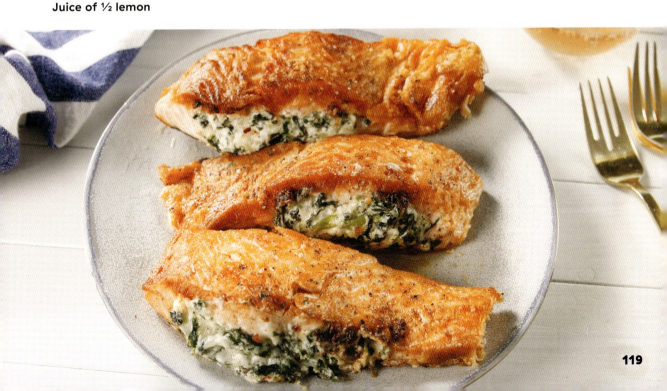

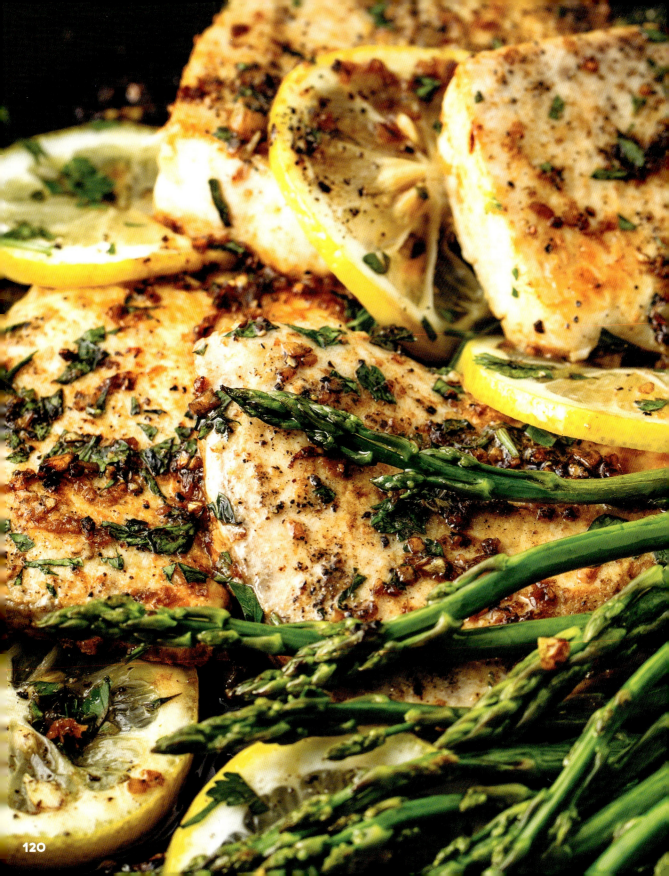

GARLICKY LEMON MAHI-MAHI

TOTAL TIME: 20 MIN / SERVES 4

Unsure of mahi-mahi? It's a white-fleshed fish with a super mild flavor. (You've probably eaten it in fish tacos.) Cod is a great sub.

- 3 tablespoons butter, divided
- 1 tablespoon extra-virgin olive oil
- 4 (4-ounce) mahi-mahi fillets
- Kosher salt
- Freshly ground black pepper
- 3 cloves garlic, minced
- Zest and juice of 1 lemon
- 1 tablespoon freshly chopped parsley, plus more for garnish

1 In a large skillet over medium heat, melt 1 tablespoon butter and olive oil. Add mahi-mahi and season with salt and pepper. Cook until golden, 3 minutes per side. Transfer to a plate.

2 To skillet, add remaining 2 tablespoons butter. Once melted, add garlic and cook until fragrant, 1 minute, then stir in lemon zest and juice and parsley. Return mahi-mahi fillets to skillet and spoon sauce over fillets.

3 Garnish with more parsley before serving.

Nutrition (per serving): 200 calories, 21 g protein, 0 g carbohydrates, 0 g fiber, 0 g sugar, 13 g fat, 6 g saturated fat, 180 mg sodium

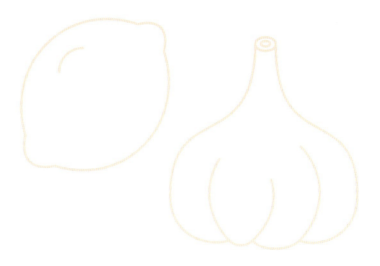

LEMON BUTTER BAKED TILAPIA

TOTAL TIME: 20 MIN / SERVES 4

If tilapia isn't your favorite, this recipe works with cod, salmon, or even shrimp.

4 tilapia filets

Kosher salt

Freshly ground black pepper

5 tablespoons butter, melted

2 cloves garlic, minced

¼ teaspoon red pepper flakes

Juice and zest of ½ lemon

1 lemon, sliced into rounds

1. Preheat oven to 400°. Season tilapia with salt and pepper and place on a small baking sheet.

2. Mix together butter, garlic, red pepper flakes, lemon juice, and zest then pour over tilapia. Place lemon rounds on top and around tilapia.

3. Bake tilapia for 10 to 12 minutes or until fish is fork tender.

Nutrition (per serving): 220 calories, 21 g protein, 1 g carbohydrates, 0 g fiber, 0 g sugar, 15 g fat, 10 g saturated fat, 170 mg sodium

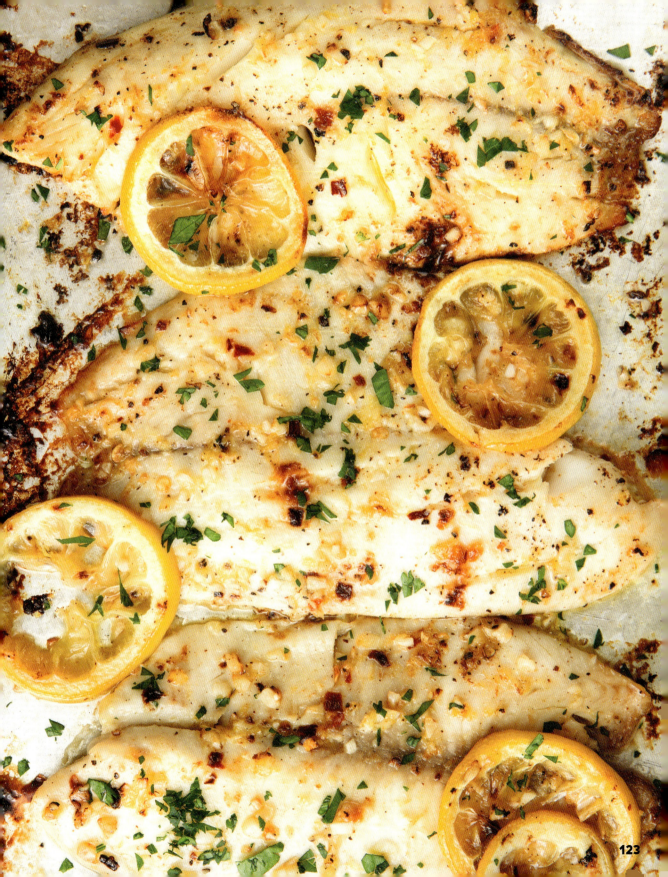

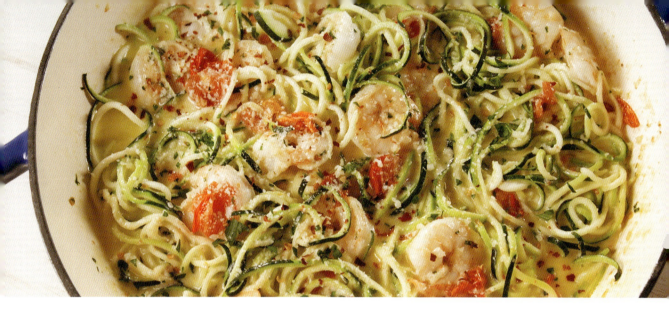

GARLICKY SHRIMP ZUCCHINI PASTA

TOTAL TIME: 15 MIN / SERVES 3 TO 4

We used to be like "Ugh" when we saw a recipe that called for zoodles, but now they're so available at grocery stores we've kind of fallen in love. When tossed with a light garlicky cream sauce, they're absolute gold.

- 3 tablespoons butter, divided
- 1 pound medium or large shrimp, peeled and deveined
- Kosher salt
- Freshly ground black pepper
- 3 cloves garlic, minced
- ¾ cup heavy cream
- ½ cup grated Parmesan
- 1 cup halved cherry tomatoes
- 3 tablespoons freshly chopped parsley
- 3 large zucchinis, spiralized (or about 4 cups zoodles)

1. In a large skillet over medium heat, melt 1 tablespoon butter. Add shrimp and season with salt and pepper. Cook until shrimp is pink and opaque, about 2 minutes per side. Transfer shrimp to a plate. (Keep juices in skillet.)

2. Melt remaining butter in skillet then stir in garlic. Cook until fragrant, about 1 minute, then whisk in heavy cream. Bring to simmer, then stir in Parmesan, tomatoes, and parsley. Simmer until tomatoes have softened and mixture has thickened slightly, about 3 minutes.

3. Return shrimp to skillet and add zucchini noodles. Toss to combine and serve immediately.

Nutrition (per serving): 410 calories, 24 g protein, 13 g carbohydrates, 3 g fiber, 7 g sugar, 30 g fat, 18 g saturated fat, 910 mg sodium

PESTO SHRIMP SKEWERS WITH CAULIFLOWER MASH

TOTAL TIME: 40 MIN / SERVES 4

This flavorful shrimp also tastes great topped on zoodles or stuffed in lettuce wraps.

1 large head cauliflower, cut into small florets
Kosher salt
1 clove garlic, grated
½ cup white wine
½ cup heavy cream
¼ cup freshly grated Parmesan
3 tablespoons butter
1 pound extra-large shrimp, peeled and deveined
Bamboo skewers, soaked in water
Extra-virgin olive oil, for drizzling
Freshly ground black pepper
1 cup pesto
¼ cup chopped fresh basil for garnish

1 Fill an 8-quart pot with cool water and cauliflower florets. Cover pot and bring to a boil. Season with salt and simmer until tender, 16 to 18 minutes. (Smaller florets will speed up this step.)

2 Drain cauliflower in a colander and transfer back to pot over medium heat. Add garlic, white wine, and 1 cup water, then season with salt. Stir and cover pot, then simmer for 5 minutes. Turn off heat and add cream, then smash with a potato masher until smooth. Fold in Parmesan and butter just before serving.

3 Preheat grill or grill pan on medium-high. Thread shrimp onto skewers. Drizzle with olive oil and season with salt and pepper. Grill shrimp until lightly charred, 2 to 3 minutes on each side.

4 Serve shrimp skewers over a bed of cauliflower mash. Drizzle pesto over shrimp and garnish with fresh basil.

Nutrition (per serving): 600 calories, 29 g protein, 15 g carbohydrates, 5 g fiber, 5 g sugar, 45 g fat, 13 g saturated fat, 1320 mg sodium

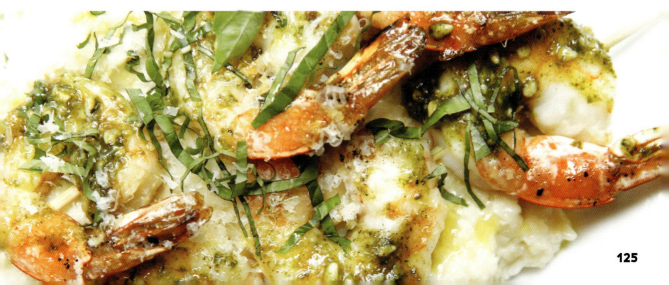

PERFECT BAKED COD

TOTAL TIME: 20 MIN / SERVES 4

If you're afraid of cooking seafood at home, cod is for you: It cooks quickly, is basically impossible to overcook, and you can flavor it however you want.

4 cod filets, about 1" thick
Kosher salt
Freshly ground black pepper
4 tablespoons extra-virgin olive oil, plus more for baking dish
1 cup cherry tomatoes
1 lemon, sliced, plus more for garnish
2 garlic cloves, smashed but not peeled
2 sprigs thyme
2 tablespoons freshly chopped parsley, for garnish

1. Preheat the oven to 400° and pat cod filets with a paper towel until dry. Season all over with salt and pepper.

2. In a medium bowl, combine olive oil, cherry tomatoes, lemon slices, garlic, and thyme.

3. Brush a baking dish with olive oil. Pour tomato-oil mixture into dish, then nestle in cod.

4. Bake until fish is opaque and flakes easily with a fork, about 15 minutes.

5. Serve garnished with parsley, more lemon juice, and the pan sauce.

Nutrition (per serving): 320 calories, 41 g protein, 1 g carbohydrates, 0 g fiber, 1 g sugar, 16 g fat, 2.5 g saturated fat, 125 mg sodium

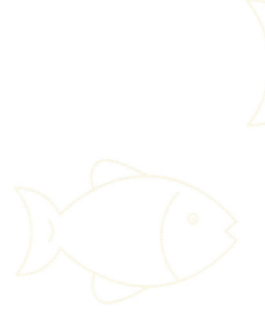

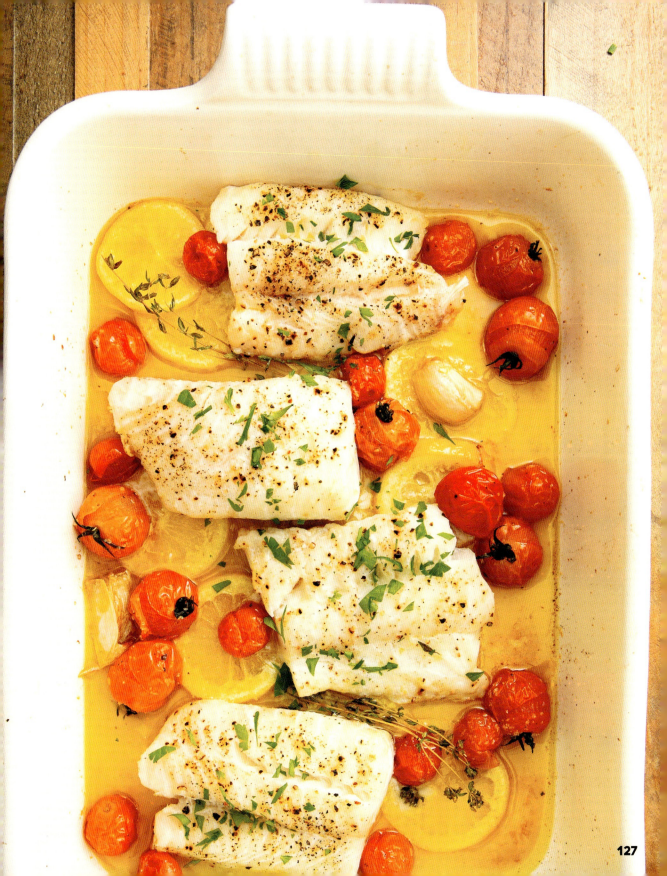

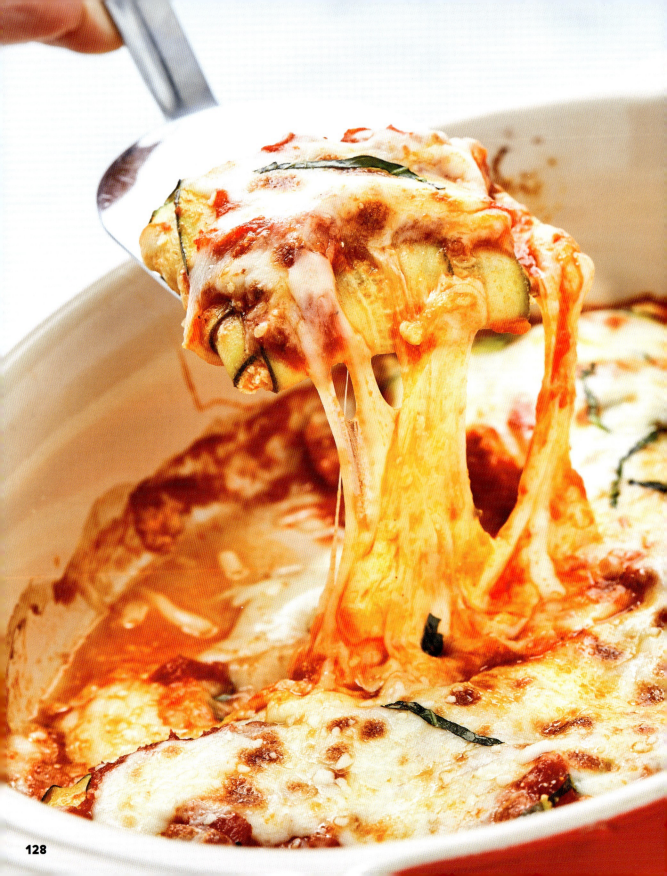

ZUCCHINI RAVIOLI

TOTAL TIME: 50 MIN / SERVES 8

Zucchini noodles can stand in for SO much more than spaghetti. This brilliant hack doesn't require a spiralizer; all you need is a vegetable peeler.

Extra-virgin olive oil, for baking dish

4 medium zucchinis

2 cups ricotta

½ cup finely grated Parmesan, plus more for garnish

1 large egg, lightly beaten

¼ cup thinly sliced basil, divided

1 clove garlic, minced

Kosher salt

Freshly ground black pepper

1½ cups marinara sauce

½ cup shredded mozzarella

1 Preheat oven to 375° and grease a large baking dish with olive oil.

2 Make the noodles: Slice 2 sides of each zucchini lengthwise to create 2 flat sides. Using a vegetable peeler, slice each zucchini into thin flat strips, peeling until you reach the center. These are your "noodles."

3 Make the filling: In a medium bowl, combine ricotta, Parmesan, egg, 2 tablespoons basil, and garlic and season with salt and pepper.

4 Assemble the ravioli: Lay 2 strips of zucchini noodles so that they overlap lengthwise. Lay 2 more noodles on top, perpendicular to the first strips. You should end up with a "T" shape. Spoon about 1 tablespoon of filling in the center of the zucchini. Bring the ends of the strips together to fold over the center, working one side at a time. Turn the ravioli over and place in the baking dish seam-side down. Repeat with remaining zucchini and filling. Pour marinara around the zucchini and top ravioli with mozzarella.

5 Bake until zucchini noodles are "al dente" and the cheese is melted and starting to brown on top; 25 to 30 minutes.

6 Top with remaining basil and garnish with Parmesan before serving.

Nutrition (per serving): 220 calories, 17 g protein, 11 g carbohydrates, 2 g fiber, 3 g sugar, 12 g fat, 7 g saturated fat, 500 mg sodium

CAPRESE STUFFED AVOCADOS

TOTAL TIME: 10 MIN / SERVES 4

Caprese salad is our go-to dish all summer, so you can find us adding the tomatoes, mozz, basil trio to pretty much everything.

2 avocados, pitted
½ cup cherry tomatoes, halved
½ cup chopped fresh mozzarella
1 teaspoon Italian seasoning
1 tablespoon balsamic vinegar
2 tablespoons extra-virgin olive oil
Kosher salt
Freshly ground black pepper
Basil, for garnish

1. Scoop out avocados, leaving a small border. Dice avocado flesh and set aside.
2. In a large bowl, toss diced avocado with tomatoes, mozzarella, Italian seasoning, balsamic, and olive oil. Season with salt and pepper.
3. Divide salad among 4 avocado halves and garnish with basil.

Nutrition (per serving): 200 calories, 6 g protein, 10 g carbohydrates, 7 g fiber, 2 g sugar, 17 g fat, 3.5 g saturated fat, 95 mg sodium

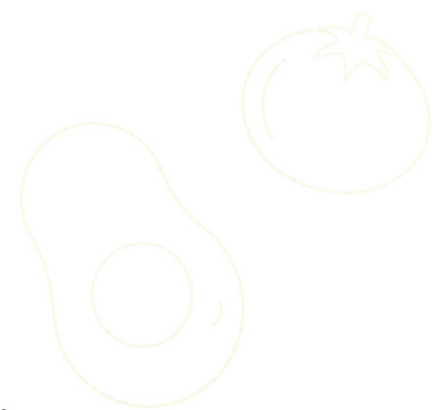

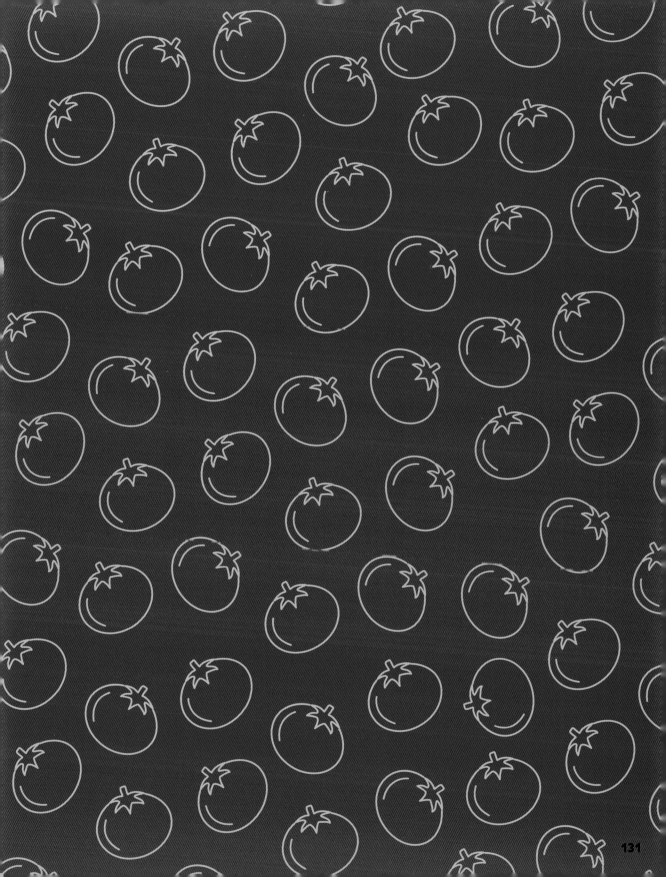

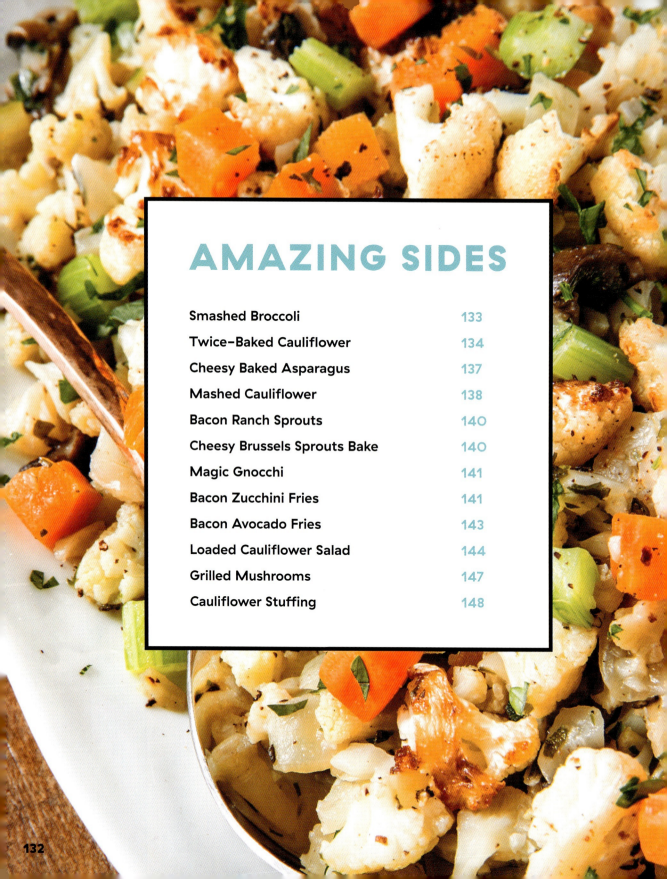

AMAZING SIDES

Smashed Broccoli	**133**
Twice-Baked Cauliflower	**134**
Cheesy Baked Asparagus	**137**
Mashed Cauliflower	**138**
Bacon Ranch Sprouts	**140**
Cheesy Brussels Sprouts Bake	**140**
Magic Gnocchi	**141**
Bacon Zucchini Fries	**141**
Bacon Avocado Fries	**143**
Loaded Cauliflower Salad	**144**
Grilled Mushrooms	**147**
Cauliflower Stuffing	**148**

SMASHED BROCCOLI

TOTAL TIME: 15 MIN / SERVES 4 TO 6

Forget roasted or steamed broccoli—smashed broccoli is where the flavor is at.

1 large head broccoli, cut into florets

Kosher salt

Extra-virgin olive oil, for frying

2 garlic cloves, smashed

Lemon wedges, for serving

1 cup grated Parmesan

Flaky sea salt, for serving

Crushed red pepper, for serving

1. Prepare a large ice bath in a large bowl or pot. In a large pot of boiling salted water, blanch broccoli until bright green and just tender, about 2 minutes. Drain broccoli then immediately transfer to ice bath. Drain broccoli again and pat dry with paper towels.

2. On a large cutting board or clean working surface, use the back of a mason jar (or small glass), to smash broccoli. (Don't press down so hard that the florets completely fall apart.)

3. In a large skillet over medium heat, pour in just enough olive oil to coat the bottom of the skillet and heat until olive oil is shimmering. Add broccoli and garlic in an even layer and cook, without moving, until the bottom of the broccoli is crispy and golden, about 3 minutes. Flip and cook until crispy on other side, another 2 minutes.

4. Remove broccoli and garlic from skillet and transfer broccoli to a paper towel–lined plate to drain. (Discard garlic—it's already done its job flavoring the olive oil!) Work in batches to cook and drain remaining broccoli.

5. Immediately plate the broccoli, squeeze lemon juice over broccoli and sprinkle with Parmesan, flaky sea salt, and red pepper flakes.

Nutrition (per serving): 90 calories, 8 g protein, 8 g carbohydrates, 3 g fiber, 2 g sugar, 4 g fat, 2.5 g saturated fat, 240 mg sodium

TWICE-BAKED CAULIFLOWER

TOTAL TIME: 40 MIN / SERVES 4

All the beauty of a twice-baked potato in a keto-friendly cauliflower form.

1 large head cauliflower, chopped into florets

½ cup sour cream, plus more for garnish

1 tablespoon butter

¾ cup shredded cheddar, divided

Kosher salt

Freshly ground black pepper

2 tablespoons finely chopped chives

4 crumbled, cooked bacon slices (optional)

1. Preheat oven to 350°. Fill a large pot with 3" of water and add a steamer insert. Bring water to a boil over high heat. Add cauliflower and cover with lid. Steam until very tender, 8 to 10 minutes.

2. Transfer steamed cauliflower to a bowl then use a potato masher to mash cauliflower. Add sour cream, butter, and ½ cup cheese, stirring until butter is melted. Season with salt and pepper.

3. Spread cauliflower into an 8"-x-8" baking dish. Top with remaining ¼ cup cheese. Bake until top is golden, 20 to 25 minutes.

4. Garnish with sour cream, chives, and bacon before serving.

Nutrition (per serving): 210 calories, 10 g protein, 11 g carbohydrates, 4 g fiber, 5 g sugar, 15 g fat, 9 g saturated fat, 240 mg sodium

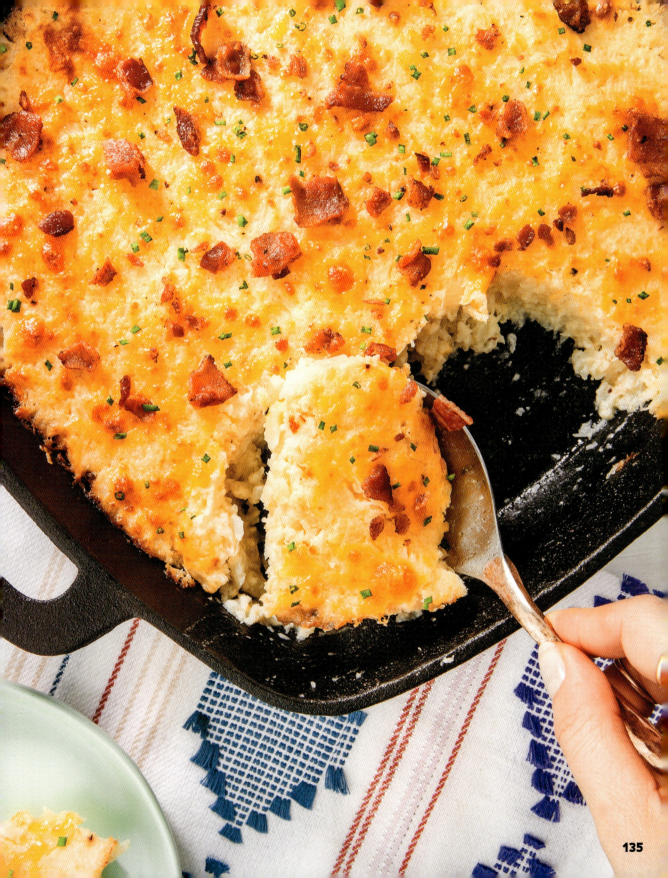

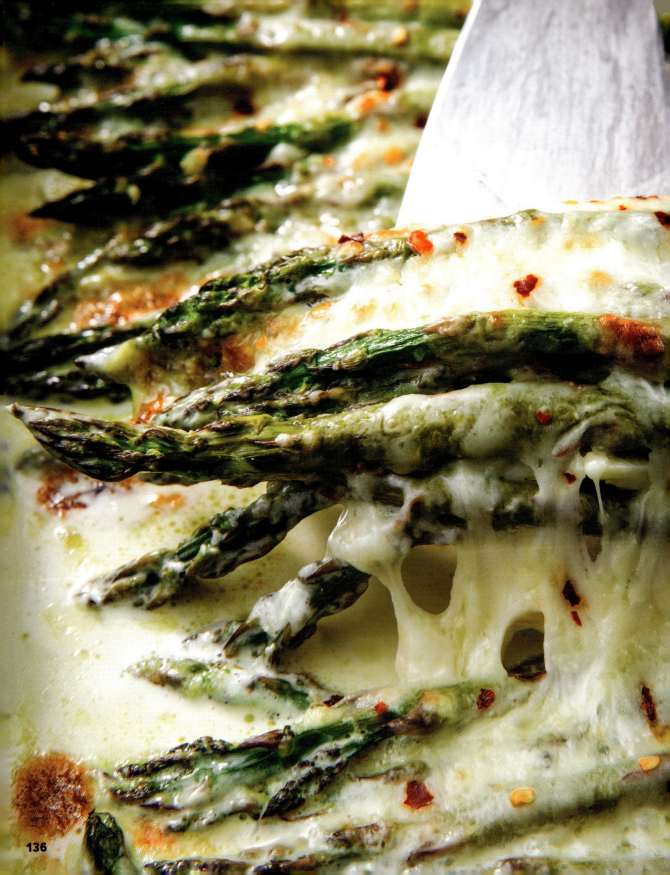

CHEESY BAKED ASPARAGUS

TOTAL TIME: 35 MIN / SERVES 6

Our favorite way to prep asparagus? Top it with garlic, a little cream, Parmesan, and mozzarella and bake until the cheese is so bubbly and golden you can't wait to dig in.

2 pounds asparagus, stalks trimmed

¾ cup heavy cream

3 cloves garlic, minced

Kosher salt

Freshly ground black pepper

1 cup freshly grated Parmesan

1 cup shredded mozzarella

Red pepper flakes, for garnish (optional)

1. Preheat oven to 400°. Place asparagus in a 13"-x-9" baking dish and pour over heavy cream and scatter with garlic. Generously season with salt and pepper, then sprinkle with Parmesan and mozzarella.

2. Bake until cheese is golden and melty and asparagus is tender, about 25 minutes.

3. Heat broiler and broil until cheese is bubbly and golden, 2 minutes. Garnish with red pepper flakes, if using, before serving.

Nutrition (per serving): 250 calories, 14 g protein, 8 g carbohydrates, 3 g fiber, 3 g sugar, 19 g fat, 11 g saturated fat, 340 mg sodium

MASHED CAULIFLOWER

TOTAL TIME: 25 MIN / SERVES 6 TO 8

The perfect low-carb substitute for mashed potatoes. The secret to making it so smooth and creamy? CREAM CHEESE!

2 medium heads cauliflower, cut into florets

6 ounces cream cheese, softened

⅓ cup milk, plus more if needed for good consistency

Kosher salt

Freshly ground black pepper

Chopped chives, for garnish

Butter, for serving

1. Bring a large pot of water to a boil over high heat. Add cauliflower florets and cook until tender, 10 minutes. Drain well, pressing with paper towels or a clean dish towel to remove as much excess water as possible.

2. Return cauliflower to pot and mash it with a potato masher until smooth and no large chunks remain.

3. Stir in cream cheese and milk. Season with salt and pepper and mash until completely combined and creamy. (Add a couple tablespoons more milk until you reach desired consistency.)

4. Before serving, garnish with chives, season with more pepper, and top with a pat of butter.

Nutrition (per serving): 110 calories, 4 g protein, 9 g carbohydrates, 3 g fiber, 4 g sugar, 8 g fat, 4.5 g saturated fat, 115 mg sodium

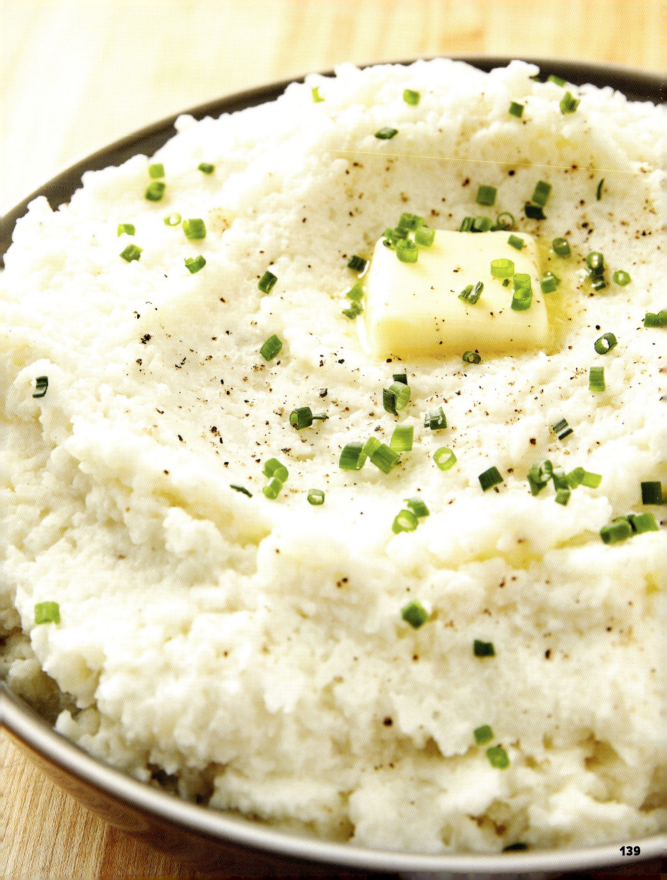

BACON RANCH SPROUTS

TOTAL TIME: 45 MIN / SERVES 4 TO 6

If you put ranch on everything (so...all of us), you need these sprouts.

1 pound Brussels sprouts, trimmed and halved

1 tablespoon olive oil

3 cloves garlic, minced

1 teaspoon dried oregano

½ teaspoon paprika

Kosher salt

Freshly ground black pepper

8 slices bacon, chopped

Ranch dressing, for drizzling

Freshly grated Parmesan, for sprinkling

1. Preheat oven to 425°. On a large baking sheet, toss Brussels sprouts with olive oil, garlic, oregano, and paprika then season with salt and pepper. Scatter bacon pieces on the pan.

2. Bake until sprouts are tender and charred, 30 minutes.

3. Drizzle with ranch dressing and sprinkle with Parmesan. Serve warm.

Nutrition (per serving): 100 calories, 6 g protein, 7 g carbohydrates, 3 g fiber, 2 g sugar, 6 g fat, 1.5 g saturated fat, 160 mg sodium

CHEESY BRUSSELS SPROUTS BAKE

TOTAL TIME: 35 MIN / SERVES 6

The one side dish that will make all your guests freak out (and run for seconds).

5 slices bacon

3 tablespoons butter

2 small shallots, minced

2 pounds Brussels sprouts, halved

Kosher salt

½ teaspoon cayenne pepper

¾ cup heavy cream

½ cup shredded sharp white cheddar

½ cup shredded Gruyère

1. Preheat oven to 375°. In a large oven-safe skillet over medium heat, cook bacon until crispy, 8 minutes. Drain on a paper towel-lined plate, then chop it. Discard bacon fat.

2. Return skillet to medium heat and melt butter. Add shallots and Brussels sprouts and season with salt and cayenne. Cook, stirring occasionally, until tender, about 10 minutes.

3. Remove from heat and drizzle with heavy cream, then top with both cheeses and bacon pieces.

4. Bake until cheese is bubbly, 12 to 15 minutes. (If your cheese isn't golden, switch oven to broil and broil 1 minute.)

Nutrition (per serving): 320 calories, 13 g protein, 15 g carbohydrates, 6 g fiber, 3 g sugar, 25 g fat, 15 g saturated fat, 280 mg sodium

MAGIC GNOCCHI

TOTAL TIME: 35 MIN / SERVES 4

What makes this gnocchi so magical? For starters, it's made of mozzarella and egg yolks.

2 cups shredded mozzarella
3 egg yolks
½ teaspoon Italian seasoning
Kosher salt
Freshly ground black pepper
8 slices bacon, chopped
2 cups baby spinach
Freshly grated Parmesan, for garnish

1. Melt mozzarella in microwave for 1 minute on high. Add egg yolks, one at a time, until completely incorporated. Stir in Italian seasoning and season with salt and pepper. Divide dough into 4 balls and refrigerate until firm, 10 minutes.
2. Roll out each ball into long logs and slice into "gnocchi."
3. In a large pot of salted boiling water, cook gnocchi 2 minutes. Drain and return to pot.
4. In a large skillet over medium heat, cook bacon until crispy, 8 minutes. Drain fat and add spinach and gnocchi. Cook until golden, 2 minutes more, then garnish with Parmesan before serving.

Nutrition (per serving): 290 calories, 22 g protein, 4 g carbohydrates, 1 g fiber, 0 g sugar, 20 g fat, 9 g saturated fat, 610 mg sodium

BACON ZUCCHINI FRIES

TOTAL TIME: 25 MIN / SERVES 8

Because anything wrapped in bacon is 1,000 times better.

Cooking spray
4 zucchinis, cut lengthwise into 4 wedges each
16 strips bacon
Ranch dressing, for serving

1. Preheat oven to 425° and spray a baking sheet with cooking spray. Wrap each zucchini wedge in bacon and place on baking sheet.
2. Bake until the bacon is cooked through and crispy, 35 minutes. Serve with ranch.

Nutrition (per serving): 90 calories, 6 g protein, 3 g carbohydrates, 1 g fiber, 2 g sugar, 6 g fat, 2 g saturated fat, 230 mg sodium

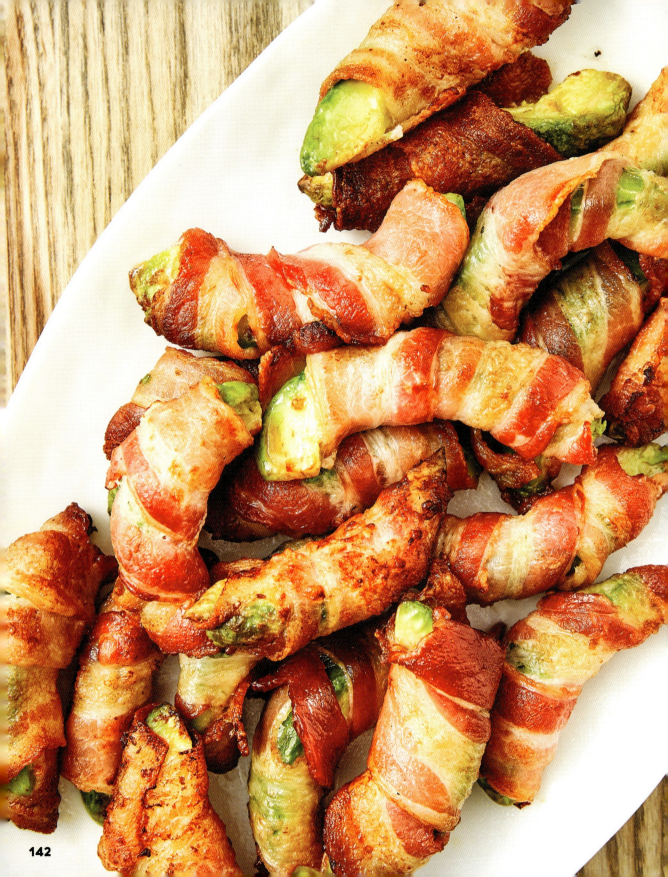

BACON AVOCADO FRIES

TOTAL TIME: 30 MIN / SERVES 12

These low-carb "fries" turn a regular slice of avocado into something extraordinary—and it won't ruin your diet.

3 avocados, pitted and peeled

12 thin strips bacon

¼ cup ranch dressing

1. Preheat oven to 425°. Slice each avocado into 4 equally sized wedges. Wrap each wedge in bacon, cutting bacon if needed. Place all 12 wedges on a baking sheet, seam-side down.

2. Bake until bacon is cooked through and crispy, 12 to 15 minutes.

3. Serve with ranch.

Nutrition (per serving): 120 calories, 4 g protein, 3 g carbohydrates, 2 g fiber, 0 g sugar, 11 g fat, 2 g saturated fat, 190 mg sodium

LOADED CAULIFLOWER SALAD

TOTAL TIME: 45 MIN / SERVES 4

Like your favorite loaded potato salad, this one's filled with plenty of bacon and cheese.

1 large head cauliflower, cut into florets
6 slices bacon
½ cup sour cream
¼ cup mayonnaise
1 tablespoon lemon juice
½ teaspoon garlic powder
Kosher salt
Freshly ground black pepper
1½ cups shredded cheddar
¼ cup finely chopped chives

1. In a large skillet, bring about ¼" water to boil. Add cauliflower, cover pan, and steam until tender, about 4 minutes. Drain and let cool while you prep other ingredients.

2. In a large skillet over medium heat, cook bacon until crispy, about 3 minutes per side. Transfer to a paper towel–lined plate to drain, then chop into small pieces.

3. In a large bowl, whisk together sour cream, mayonnaise, lemon juice, and garlic powder. Add cauliflower and toss gently. Season with salt and pepper, then fold in bacon, cheddar, and chives. Serve warm or at room temperature.

Nutrition (per serving): 440 calories, 19 g protein, 13 g carbohydrates, 4 g fiber, 5 g sugar, 35 g fat, 15 g saturated fat, 570 mg sodium

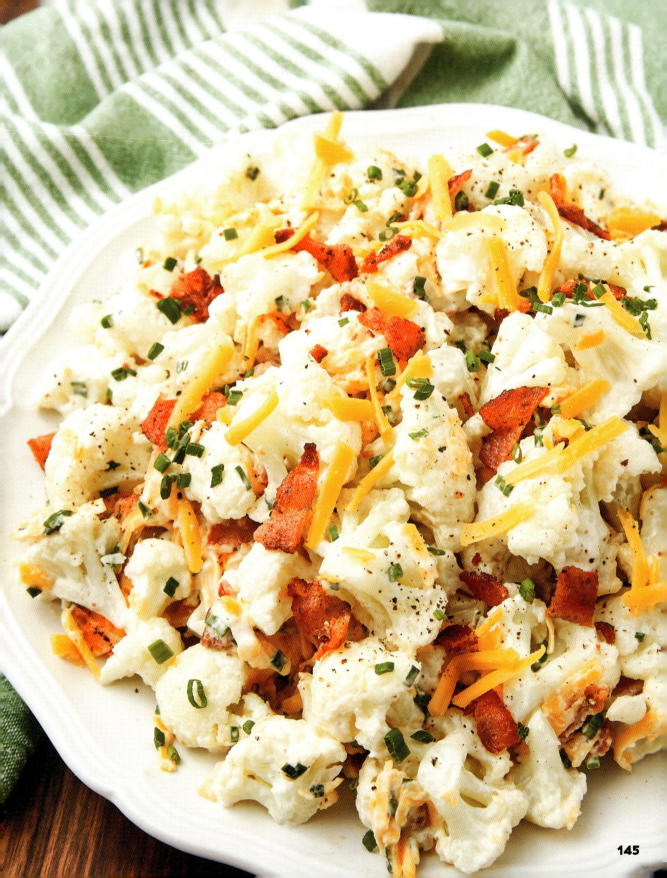

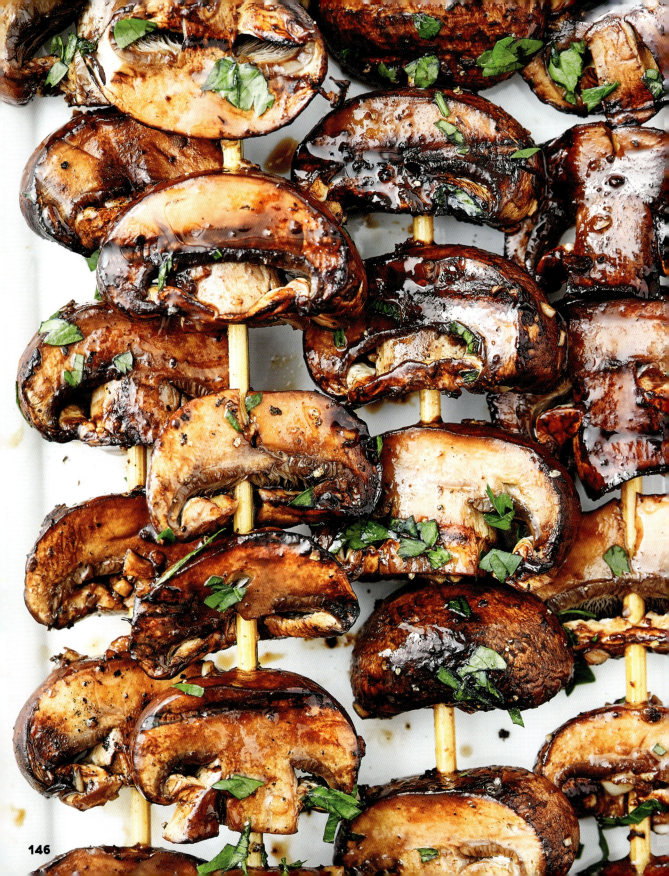

GRILLED MUSHROOMS

TOTAL TIME: 35 MIN / SERVES 4

Mushrooms can get sidelined at a barbecue as the lame side for vegetarians, but when tossed in a balsamic-soy glaze, they'll get all the attention.

- ¼ cup balsamic vinegar
- 2 tablespoons low-sodium soy sauce
- 2 cloves garlic, minced
- Freshly ground black pepper
- 1 pound cremini mushrooms, sliced ½" thick
- Freshly chopped parsley, for garnish

1. In a large bowl, whisk together balsamic, soy sauce, garlic, and pepper. Add mushrooms and marinate 20 minutes.
2. Heat grill to medium-high. Skewer mushrooms and grill 2 to 3 minutes per side.
3. Garnish with parsley before serving.

Nutrition (per serving): 45 calories, 3 g protein, 9 g carbohydrates, 1 g fiber, 4 g sugar, 0 g fat, 0 g saturated fat, 280 mg sodium

CAULIFLOWER STUFFING

TOTAL TIME: 30 MIN / SERVES 6

Cauliflower takes the place of bread crumbs in the low-carb holiday side of your dreams.

4 tablespoons butter

1 onion, chopped

2 large carrots, peeled and chopped

2 celery stalks, chopped or thinly sliced

1 small head cauliflower, chopped

1 cup chopped mushrooms

Kosher salt

Freshly ground black pepper

¼ cup chopped fresh parsley

2 tablespoons chopped fresh rosemary

1 tablespoon chopped fresh sage (or 1 teaspoon ground sage)

½ cup vegetable or chicken broth

1. In a large skillet over medium heat, melt butter. Add onion, carrot, and celery and cook until soft, 7 to 8 minutes.

2. Add cauliflower and mushrooms and season with salt and pepper. Cook until tender, 8 to 10 minutes more.

3. Add parsley, rosemary, and sage and stir until combined, then pour in broth and cover with a lid. Cook covered, until totally tender and liquid is absorbed, 15 minutes.

Nutrition (per serving): 90 calories, 6 g protein, 3 g carbohydrates, 1 g fiber, 2 g sugar, 6 g fat, 2 g saturated fat, 230 mg sodium

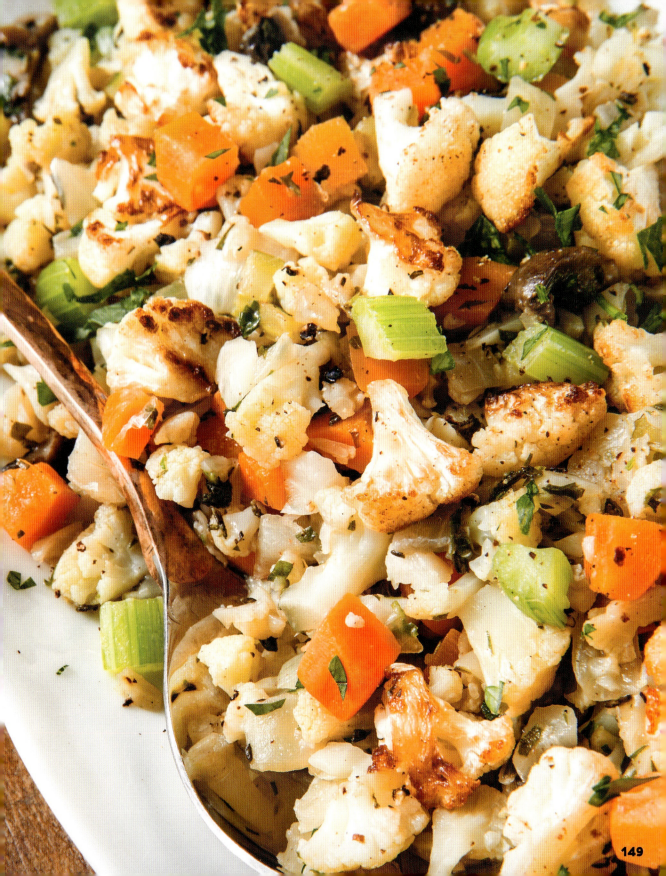

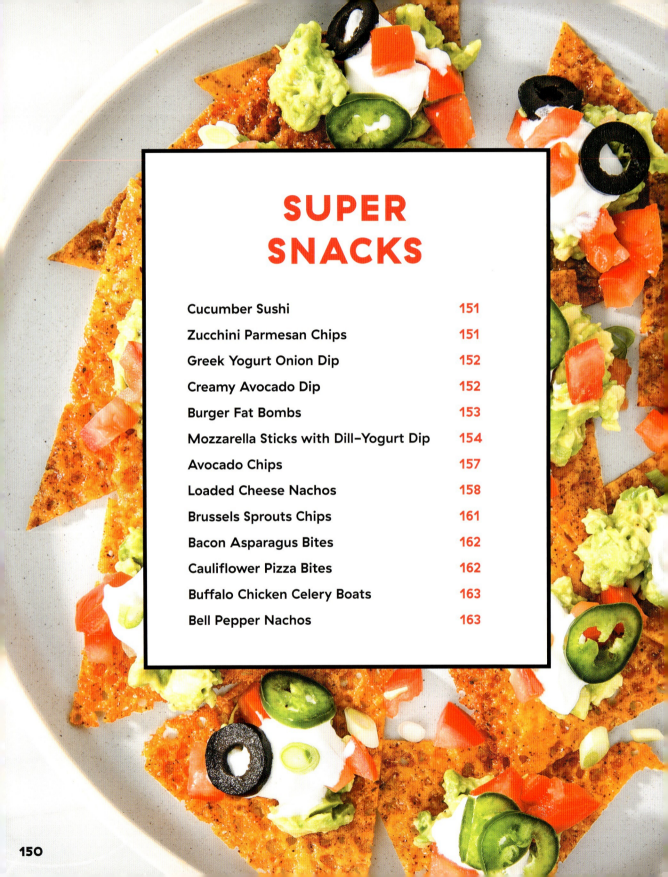

SUPER SNACKS

Cucumber Sushi	151
Zucchini Parmesan Chips	151
Greek Yogurt Onion Dip	152
Creamy Avocado Dip	152
Burger Fat Bombs	153
Mozzarella Sticks with Dill-Yogurt Dip	154
Avocado Chips	157
Loaded Cheese Nachos	158
Brussels Sprouts Chips	161
Bacon Asparagus Bites	162
Cauliflower Pizza Bites	162
Buffalo Chicken Celery Boats	163
Bell Pepper Nachos	163

CUCUMBER SUSHI

TOTAL TIME: 20 MIN / SERVES 4

We know it's not real sushi, but we love it just the same.

FOR THE SUSHI:

2 medium cucumbers, chopped in half

¼ avocado, peeled and thinly sliced

½ red bell pepper, thinly sliced

½ yellow bell pepper, thinly sliced

2 small carrots, thinly sliced

FOR THE DIPPING SAUCE:

⅓ cup mayonnaise

1 tablespoon sriracha

1 teaspoon soy sauce

1. Using a small spoon, remove seeds from center of cucumbers until they are completely hollow.
2. Press avocado slices deep into the center of cucumber, using a butter knife. Next, slide in bell peppers and carrots until the cucumber is completely full of veggies.
3. Make dipping sauce: Combine mayo, sriracha, and soy sauce in a small bowl. Whisk to combine.
4. Slice cucumber rounds into 1"-thick pieces and serve with dipping sauce on the side.

Nutrition (per serving): 190 calories, 1 g protein, 9 g carbohydrates, 3 g fiber, 5 g sugar, 16 g fat, 2 g saturated fat, 240 mg sodium

ZUCCHINI PARMESAN CHIPS

TOTAL TIME: 35 MIN / SERVES 4

While these don't have a crunchy texture like potato chips, the salty Parmesan makes them equally satisfying.

2 large zucchinis, thinly sliced

Kosher salt

Freshly ground black pepper

1½ cups freshly grated Parmesan

Marinara sauce, for dipping

1. Preheat oven to 400° and line a baking sheet with parchment. Arrange zucchini slices on baking sheet and season with salt and pepper. Top each with Parmesan.
2. Bake until deeply golden and crisp, 20 to 25 minutes.
3. Serve with marinara sauce.

Nutrition (per serving): 160 calories, 13 g protein, 6 g carbohydrates, 1 g fiber, 4 g sugar, 9 g fat, 5 g saturated fat, 470 mg sodium

GREEK YOGURT ONION DIP

TOTAL TIME: 40 MIN / SERVES 8

A healthier alternative to one of our all-time-favorite dips.

2 tablespoons olive oil

2 onions, thinly sliced

2 teaspoons fresh thyme leaves

Kosher salt

Freshly ground black pepper

1 tablespoon apple cider vinegar

2 cups Greek yogurt

Carrot sticks, for serving

1 Heat olive oil in a medium skillet over medium heat. Add onions and thyme. Season to taste with salt and pepper. Turn down the heat to medium-low and cook, stirring occasionally, until soft and caramelized—about 20 minutes. If the onions are browning too quickly, turn down the heat and add a splash of water. When the onions are caramelized and jammy, add the vinegar. Reduce the vinegar slightly, about 1 minute, and remove from heat.

2 In a medium serving bowl, combine caramelized onions and yogurt.

3 Serve cold or at room temperature with carrot sticks.

Nutrition (per serving): 80 calories, 5 g protein, 5 g carbohydrates, 1 g fiber, 3 g sugar, 4.5 g fat, 1 g saturated fat, 20 mg sodium

CREAMY AVOCADO DIP

TOTAL TIME: 5 MIN / SERVES 4

This ultra-creamy dip is packed with protein and healthy fats.

2 ripe avocados, pitted and peeled

½ cup plain Greek yogurt

2 cloves garlic, minced

Juice of 1 lime

Kosher salt

Freshly ground black pepper

1 In a large bowl, mash avocados.

2 Add yogurt, garlic, and lime juice and season with salt and pepper.

Nutrition (per serving): 140 calories, 4 g protein, 9 g carbohydrates, 5 g fiber, 2 g sugar, 11 g fat, 2 g saturated fat, 15 mg sodium

BURGER FAT BOMBS

TOTAL TIME: 30 MIN / SERVES 20

The secret ingredient in these burger fat bombs: BUTTER. These will help keep you satisfied for way longer than your favorite fast food joint ever could.

Cooking spray, for muffin tin
1 pound ground beef
½ teaspoon garlic powder
Kosher salt
Freshly ground black pepper
2 tablespoons cold butter, cut into 20 pieces
¼ (8-ounce) block cheddar cheese, cut into 20 pieces
Lettuce leaves, for serving
Thinly sliced tomatoes, for serving
Mustard, for serving

1. Preheat oven to 375° and grease a mini muffin tin with cooking spray. In a medium bowl, season beef with garlic powder, salt, and pepper.

2. Press about 1 tablespoon of beef into the bottom of each muffin tin cup, completely covering the bottom. Place a piece of butter on top then press about 1 tablespoon of beef over the butter to completely cover.

3. Place a piece of cheese on top of meat in each cup then press remaining beef over cheese to completely cover.

4. Bake until meat is cooked through, about 15 minutes. Let cool slightly.

5. Carefully, use a metal offset spatula to release each burger from the tin. Serve with lettuce leaves, tomatoes, and mustard.

Nutrition (per serving): 80 calories, 5 g protein, 0 g carbohydrates, 0 g fiber, 0 g sugar, 7 g fat, 3 g saturated fat, 45 mg sodium

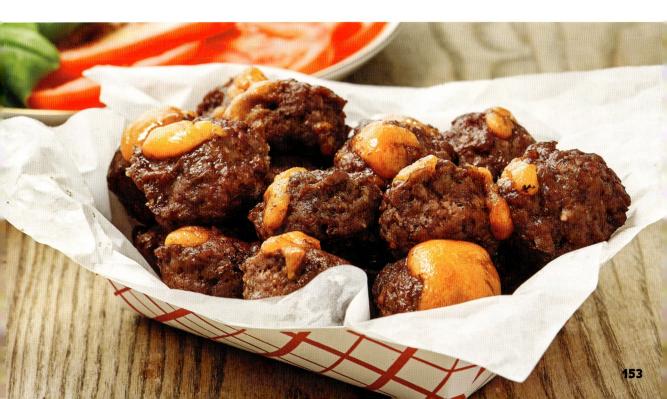

MOZZARELLA STICKS WITH DILL-YOGURT DIP

TOTAL TIME: 40 MIN / SERVES 4

Pro tip: you can also makes these with salty Halloumi cut into thin slices.

- 1 large egg
- 1 tablespoon water
- Kosher salt
- Freshly ground black pepper
- ½ cup almond flour
- ½ cup grated Parmesan
- 6 (1-ounce) sticks mozzarella string cheese
- ½ cup Greek yogurt
- 1 tablespoon white vinegar
- ½ teaspoon garlic powder
- 2 tablespoons chopped fresh dill
- 1 tablespoon chopped chives or scallions
- 2 tablespoons canola oil

1. In a small bowl, whisk together egg, and water. Season with salt and pepper.

2. Line a plate with parchment paper. In a shallow dish, mix almond flour and Parmesan until combined. Coat string cheese first in almond flour mixture, then egg, then the almond flour mixture again. Place on prepared plate. Repeat to coat all string cheese sticks. Freeze mozzarella sticks for 15 to 20 minutes.

3. Meanwhile, in a small bowl, combine yogurt, vinegar, garlic powder, dill, and chives. Refrigerate until needed.

4. In a medium skillet over medium-high heat, heat oil. In batches, cook breaded cheese until golden on each side, about 2 minutes per side.

5. Serve mozzarella sticks with yogurt sauce for dipping.

Nutrition (per serving): 340 calories, 23 g protein, 6 carbohydrates, 2 g fiber, 2 g sugar, 28 g fat, 9 g saturated fat, 550 mg sodium

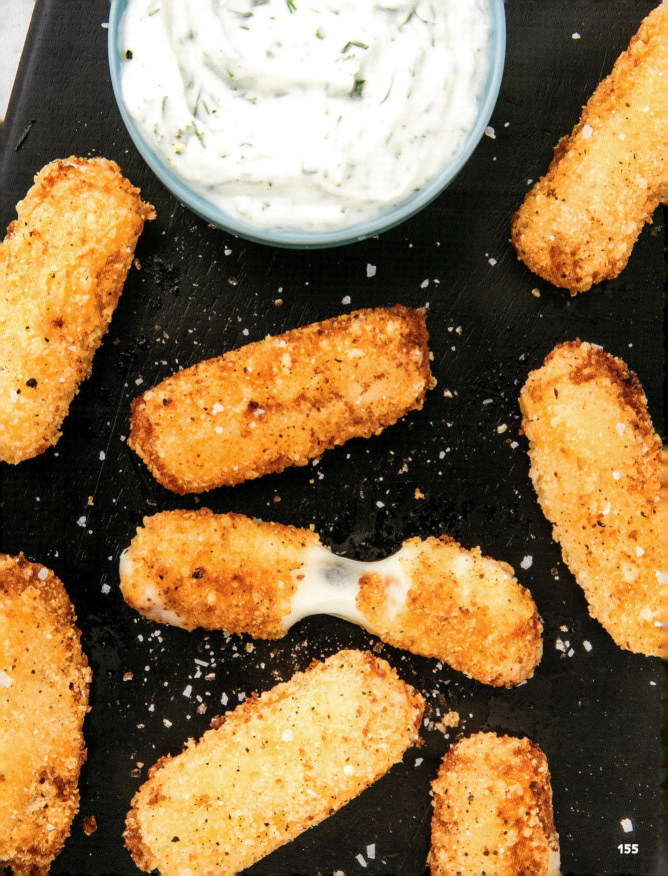

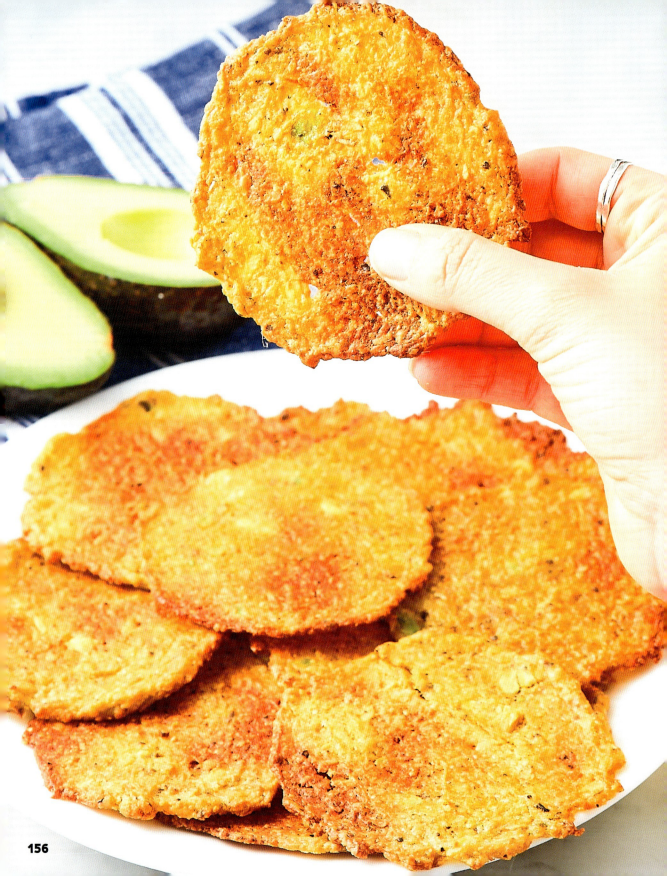

AVOCADO CHIPS

TOTAL TIME: 25 MIN / SERVES 4

Having a hard time getting your chips nice and thin? Spray the bottom of a dry measuring cup with cooking spray and press lightly to flatten the avocado mixture.

1 large ripe avocado, pitted and peeled

¾ cup freshly grated Parmesan

1 teaspoon lemon juice

½ teaspoon garlic powder

½ teaspoon Italian seasoning

Kosher salt

Freshly ground black pepper

1 Preheat oven to 325° and line a medium baking sheet with parchment paper. In a medium bowl, mash avocado with a fork until smooth. Stir in Parmesan, lemon juice, garlic powder, and Italian seasoning. Season with salt and pepper.

2 Place heaping teaspoon–sized scoops of mixture on baking sheet, leaving about 3" between each scoop. Flatten each scoop with the back of a spoon or measuring cup. Bake until crisp and golden, 15 to 18 minutes, then let cool completely. Serve at room temperature.

Nutrition (per serving): 120 calories, 7 g protein, 4 g carbohydrates, 2 g fiber, 0 g sugar, 10 g fat, 3.5 g saturated fat, 230 mg sodium

LOADED CHEESE NACHOS

TOTAL TIME: 30 MIN / SERVES 4

When the "chips" are just made of cheddar and Parm, you can eat as many as you want, right?

FOR THE CHEESE CHIPS:
2 cups shredded cheddar
¾ cup freshly grated Parmesan
2 teaspoons chili powder
½ teaspoon sweet paprika

FOR THE NACHOS:
1 avocado, halved, pitted, and diced
2 teaspoons lime juice
Kosher salt
Freshly ground black pepper
¼ cup sour cream
⅓ cup sliced black olives
1 medium tomato, chopped
2 green onions, thinly sliced
1 jalapeño, thinly sliced (optional)

1. Preheat the oven to 400° and line a rimmed half sheet pan with parchment paper. In a large bowl, mix cheeses, chili powder, and paprika until combined. Spread mixture onto sheet pan in an even layer.

2. Bake until cheese is browned and crispy to the touch, 10 to 12 minutes. Let cheese cool slightly.

3. Use kitchen shears to cut cheese into strips then cut each strip into a triangle or square. Return cheese chips to sheet pan and bake for 2 to 3 minutes more, until crispier. Let chips cool 5 to 10 minutes.

4. In a small bowl, mash the avocado with a fork. Stir in lime juice and season with salt and pepper. Spread cheese chips onto a platter. Dollop with guacamole and sour cream. Top with the olives, tomatoes, green onions, and (optional) jalapeño before serving.

Nutrition (per serving): 410 calories, 21 g protein, 9 g carbohydrates, 3 g fiber, 2 g sugar, 32 g fat, 17 g saturated fat, 680 mg sodium

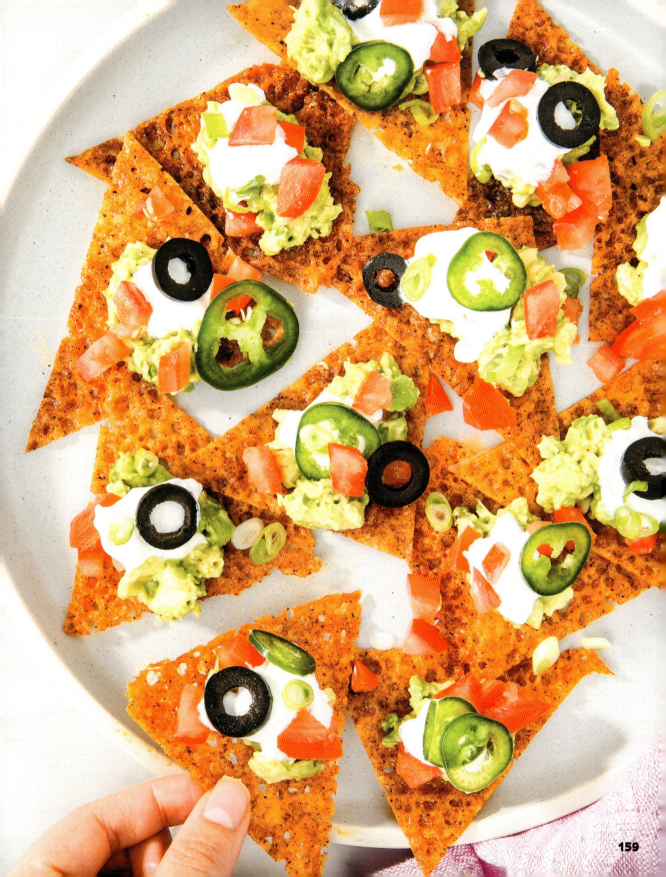

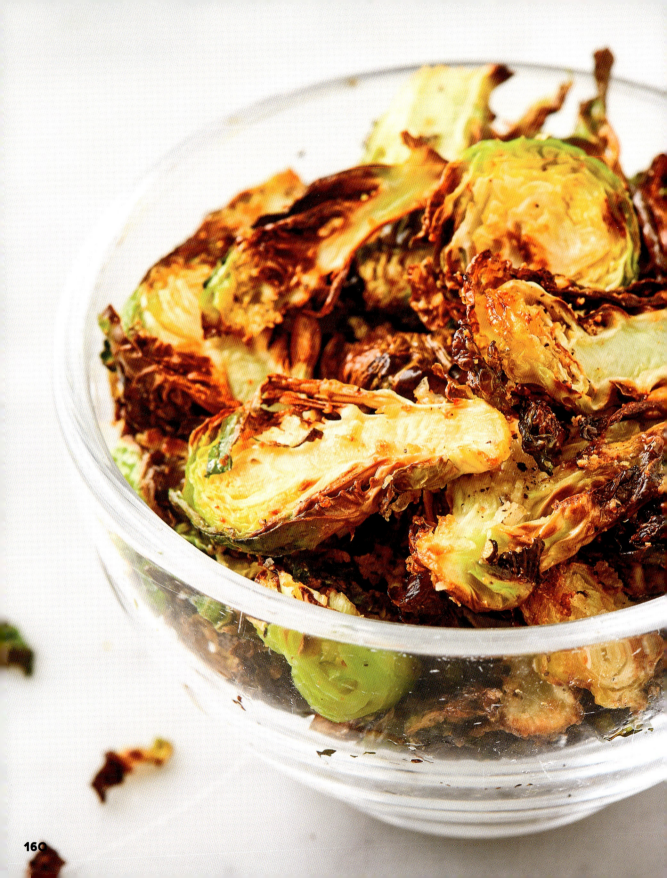

BRUSSELS SPROUTS CHIPS

TOTAL TIME: 25 MIN / SERVES 2 TO 3

All of the crunch, none of the guilt. These low-carb chips are seriously addicting.

½ pound Brussels sprouts, thinly sliced

1 tablespoon olive oil

2 tablespoons freshly grated Parmesan

1 teaspoon garlic powder

Kosher salt

Freshly ground black pepper

Caesar dressing, for dipping

1 Preheat oven to 400°. In a large bowl, toss Brussels sprouts with olive oil, Parmesan, and garlic powder and season with salt and pepper. Spread in an even layer on a medium baking sheet.

2 Bake 10 minutes, toss, and bake 8 to 10 minutes more, until crisp and golden. Serve with Caesar dressing for dipping.

Nutrition (per serving): 100 calories, 5 g protein, 8 g carbohydrates, 3 g fiber, 2 g sugar, 6 g fat, 1.5 g saturated fat, 95 mg sodium

BACON ASPARAGUS BITES

TOTAL TIME: 30 MIN / SERVES 6

Asparagus + cream cheese + bacon = yes, please.

- 6 slices bacon, cut into thirds
- 5 ounces cream cheese, softened to room temperature
- 1 garlic clove, minced
- Kosher salt
- Freshly ground black pepper
- 9 asparagus spears, trimmed and blanched

1. Preheat oven to 400° and line a medium baking sheet with parchment paper.
2. Cook bacon: In a large skillet over medium heat, cook bacon until most of the fat is cooked out, but is not crisp. Remove from pan and drain on a paper towel–lined plate.
3. In a small bowl, combine cream cheese with garlic and season with salt and pepper. Stir until combined.
4. Assemble bites: Spread about ½ tablespoon cream cheese mix onto each strip of bacon. Place asparagus in the center and roll bacon until bacon ends meet. Once all bites are made, place on prepared baking sheet and bake 5 minutes, until bacon is crisp and cream cheese is warmed through.

Nutrition (per serving): 130 calories, 5 g protein, 3 g carbohydrates, 1 g fiber, 1 g sugar, 11 g fat, 6 g saturated fat, 210 mg sodium

CAULIFLOWER PIZZA BITES

TOTAL TIME: 45 MIN / SERVES 6

Cauli crust is all the rage, and this mini version explains why.

- 1 large head cauliflower
- 2 large eggs
- 1 cup shredded mozzarella, divided
- ¼ cup freshly grated Parmesan
- 3 tablespoons finely chopped fresh basil, divided
- 1 tablespoon garlic powder
- Kosher salt
- Freshly ground black pepper
- ½ cup marinara sauce
- ¼ cup mini pepperoni slices

1. Preheat oven to 400°. Grate cauliflower on the small side of a box grater to form fine crumbs. Transfer to a large bowl.
2. Add eggs, ⅓ cup mozzarella, Parmesan, 2 tablespoons basil, and garlic powder to bowl and season with salt and pepper. Form into small patties (they will be wet) and place on a greased baking sheet. Bake until golden, 20 minutes.
3. Top each cauli patty with a thin layer of marinara, a sprinkle of the remaining mozz, and mini pepperoni and bake until cheese melts and pepperoni crisps, 5 to 7 minutes more.
4. Garnish with remaining basil before serving.

Nutrition (per serving): 430 calories, 22 g protein, 11 g carbohydrates, 3 g fiber, 3 g sugar, 33 g fat, 15 g saturated fat, 1320 mg sodium

BUFFALO CHICKEN CELERY BOATS

TOTAL TIME: 15 MIN / SERVES 2 TO 4

If you love the flavor of buffalo wings, these will become your new favorite 3 p.m. fix. Not a ranch fan? Skip it.

- ⅓ cup Frank's hot sauce
- 2 tablespoons mayonnaise
- Kosher salt
- Freshly ground black pepper
- 2 cups shredded rotisserie chicken
- 4 stalks celery, cut into 3" pieces
- ⅓ cup crumbled blue cheese
- Ranch, for drizzling
- Chives, for garnish

1. In a medium bowl, whisk together hot sauce and mayo and season with salt and pepper. Pour over shredded chicken and mix to combine. Spoon chicken mixture into celery boats.
2. Top with blue cheese, drizzle with ranch and garnish with chives.

Nutrition (per serving): 210 calories, 8 g protein, 2 g carbohydrates, 1 g fiber, 1 g sugar, 19 g fat, 6 g saturated fat, 830 mg sodium

BELL PEPPER NACHOS

TOTAL TIME: 40 MIN / SERVES 6

Who knew bell peppers were sturdy enough to make the perfect low-carb base for nachos?!

- 4 bell peppers, cut into small wedges
- 2 tablespoons extra-virgin olive oil
- ½ teaspoon ground cumin
- ½ teaspoon chili powder
- ¼ teaspoon garlic powder
- Kosher salt
- Freshly ground black pepper
- 1½ cups shredded Monterey Jack
- 1½ cups shredded cheddar
- 1 cup guacamole
- ½ cup pickled jalapeños
- 1 cup pico de gallo
- ½ cup sour cream
- 1 tablespoon milk (or water)
- Chopped fresh cilantro, for garnish
- Lime wedges, for serving

1. Preheat oven to 425° and line 2 small baking sheets with foil.
2. Divide bell peppers between baking sheets. Toss wedges on both sheets with olive oil, cumin, chili powder, and garlic powder. Season generously with salt and pepper. Lay the wedges on the baking sheets in single layers, cut-side up. Bake until the peppers are crisp-tender.
3. Top one baking sheet full of peppers with about half each of the Monterey Jack and cheddar. Top with bell peppers from the second sheet, then top with the rest of the cheese. Bake until cheese is bubbly, about 10 minutes.
4. Top bell peppers with guacamole, pickled jalapeños, and salsa. In a small bowl, whisk sour cream and milk together and drizzle over bell peppers.
5. Garnish with cilantro and serve warm with lime wedges.

Nutrition (per serving): 410 calories, 17 g protein, 13 g carbohydrates, 5 g fiber, 7g sugar, 32 g fat, 15 g saturated fat, 760 mg sodium

BREAD, BUNS & MORE

Low-Carb Sandwich Bread	165
Zucchini Taco Shells	165
Jalapeño Popper Bread	166
Burger Buns	166
Garlic Bread	167
Cloud Bread (Three Ways!)	168
Cheesy Cauli Bread	170
Broccoli Cheesy Bread	171
Cauliflower Garlic Bread	172

LOW-CARB SANDWICH BREAD

TOTAL TIME: 1 HR 10 MIN / SERVES 4

Trust us, we were skeptical at first that this would work. But turns out whipped egg whites, melted butter, and almond flour can produce an amazing slice.

6 large eggs

½ teaspoon cream of tartar

¼ cup (½ stick) butter, melted and cooled

1½ cups finely ground almond flour

1 tablespoon baking powder

½ teaspoon kosher salt

1. Preheat oven to 375° and line an 8"-x-4" loaf pan with parchment paper. Separate egg whites and egg yolks.

2. In a large bowl, combine egg whites and cream of tartar. Using a hand mixer, whip until stiff peaks form.

3. In a separate large bowl using a hand mixer, beat yolks with melted butter, almond flour, baking powder, and salt. Fold in ⅓ of the whipped egg whites until fully incorporated, then fold in the rest.

4. Pour batter into loaf pan and smooth the top. Bake for 30 minutes, or until top is slightly golden and toothpick inserted comes out clean. Let cool 30 minutes before slicing.

Nutrition (per serving): 450 calories, 19 g protein, 10 g carbohydrates, 5 g fiber, 2 g sugar, 40 g fat, 11 g saturated fat, 125 mg sodium

ZUCCHINI TACO SHELLS

TOTAL TIME: 1 HR / SERVES 6

Is there anything zucchini can't do?! Beyond pasta and sandwich bread, you can turn the squash into taco shells, too.

3 cups grated zucchini (about 3 small zucchinis)

Kosher salt

¼ cup almond flour

½ cup grated cheddar cheese

1 large egg, lightly beaten

¼ teaspoon garlic powder

Freshly ground black pepper

Toppings of choice

1. Heat oven to 400° and line a baking sheet with parchment paper. Put zucchini in a strainer and lightly salt. Let sit in the sink or over a bowl to drain as much moisture as possible, about 20 minutes.

2. In a large bowl, mix together zucchini, almond flour, cheese, egg, and garlic powder. Season with pepper.

3. Scoop ¼-cup portions of the mixture onto the baking sheet, then press each gently down until ⅛" thick.

4. Bake until the shells are lightly browned and crisp, about 25 minutes. Let cool slightly, then fill with toppings of choice.

Nutrition (per serving): 90 calories, 5 g protein, 3 g carbohydrates, 1 g fiber, 2 g sugar, 6 g fat, 2.5 g saturated fat, 75 mg sodium

JALAPEÑO POPPER BREAD

TOTAL TIME: 1 HR / SERVES 16

This low-carb recipe is so airy it doesn't totally resemble a bread, BUT, with sharp cheddar, garlic powder, jalapeños, and lots of black pepper, it's packed with so much flavor that you won't care.

Cooking spray
6 large egg whites
¾ teaspoon cream of tartar
¼ (8-ounce) block cream cheese, softened
4 large egg yolks
1 teaspoon garlic powder
¾ teaspoon kosher salt
½ cup shredded cheddar
1 jalapeño, thinly sliced

1. Preheat oven to 300°. Line a large baking sheet with parchment paper, and grease with cooking spray. In a large bowl using a hand mixer (or in the bowl of a stand mixer using the whisk attachment), beat egg whites with cream of tartar until stiff peaks form.

2. In a separate large bowl using a hand mixer, beat cream cheese, egg yolks, garlic powder, and salt until evenly incorporated. Gently fold in egg whites and cheddar.

3. Scoop ¼-cup portions onto prepared sheet, then top each with jalapeño slices. Bake until golden and puffed, about 25 minutes.

Nutrition (per serving): 50 calories, 3 g protein, 1 g carbohydrates, 0 g fiber, 0 g sugar, 3.5 g fat, 2 g saturated fat, 150 mg sodium

BURGER BUNS

TOTAL TIME: 20 MIN / SERVES 6

If you can't imagine a big, juicy burger without a bun, we've got you covered with this almond flour-based recipe.

2 cups shredded mozzarella
4 ounces cream cheese
3 large eggs
3 cups almond flour
2 teaspoons baking powder
1 teaspoon kosher salt
¼ cup (½ stick) butter, melted
Sesame seeds, for sprinkling
Dried parsley, for sprinkling

1. Preheat oven to 400° and line a baking sheet with parchment paper. In a large microwave-safe bowl, melt together mozzarella and cream cheese.

2. Add eggs and stir to combine, then add almond flour, baking powder, and salt. Form dough into 6 balls and flatten slightly then place on prepared baking sheet.

3. Brush with butter and sprinkle with sesame seeds and parsley. Bake until golden, 10 to 12 minutes.

Nutrition (per serving): 600 calories, 26 g protein, 15 g carbohydrates, 6 g fiber, 3 g sugar, 52 g fat, 15 g saturated fat, 910 mg sodium

GARLIC BREAD

TOTAL TIME: 30 MIN / SERVES 4

The secret to amazing low-carb bread? Cheese—lots of it.

- 1 cup shredded mozzarella
- ½ cup finely ground almond flour
- 2 tablespoons cream cheese
- 1 tablespoon garlic powder
- 1 tablespoon baking powder
- Kosher salt
- 1 large egg
- 1 tablespoon butter, melted
- 1 clove garlic, minced
- 1 tablespoon freshly chopped parsley
- 1 tablespoon freshly grated Parmesan
- Marinara sauce, warmed, for serving

1. Preheat oven to 400° and line a large baking sheet with parchment paper.
2. In a medium, microwave-safe bowl, add mozzarella, almond flour, cream cheese, garlic powder, baking powder, and a large pinch of salt. Microwave on high until cheeses are melted, about 1 minute. Stir in egg.
3. Shape dough into a ½"-thick oval on baking sheet.
4. In a small bowl, mix melted butter with garlic, parsley, and Parmesan. Brush mixture over top of bread.
5. Bake until golden, 15 to 17 minutes. Slice and serve with marinara sauce for dipping.

Nutrition (per serving): 250 calories, 13 g protein, 7 g carbohydrates, 2 g fiber, 1 g sugar, 20 g fat, 7 g saturated fat, 640 mg sodium

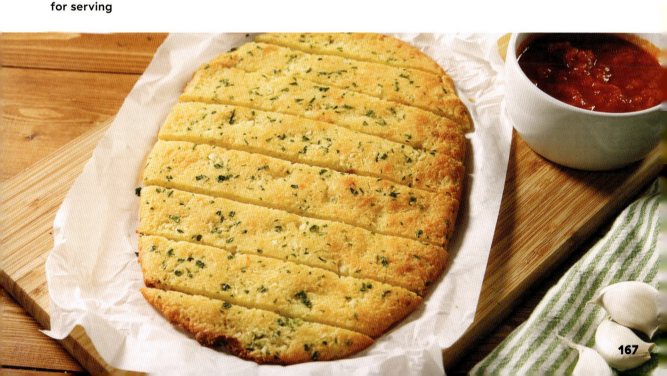

CLOUD BREAD (THREE WAYS!)

TOTAL TIME: 40 MIN / MAKES 8 PIECES

Named for its "light as a cloud" texture, this bread—basically made of just whipped egg whites—can be eaten on its own or used to make a sandwich.

3 large eggs, at room temperature

¼ teaspoon cream of tartar

Pinch of kosher salt

2 ounces cream cheese, softened

Parmesan, for garnish

1. Preheat the oven to 300° and line a large baking sheet with parchment paper.

2. Separate egg whites from yolks into 2 medium glass bowls. Add cream of tartar and salt to egg whites, then using a hand mixer, beat until stiff peaks form, 2 to 3 minutes. Add cream cheese to egg yolks, then, using a hand mixer, mix yolks and cream cheese until combined. Gently fold egg yolk mixture into egg whites.

3. Divide mixture into 8 mounds on prepared baking sheet, spacing them about 4" apart. Bake until golden, 25 to 30 minutes.

4. Immediately sprinkle each piece of bread with cheese and bake until melty, 2 to 3 minutes more. Let cool slightly.

Nutrition (per serving): 50 calories, 3 g protein, 10 g carbohydrates, 0 g fiber, 0 g sugar, 4 g fat, 2 g saturated fat, 50 mg sodium

---

PIZZA CLOUD BREAD: Stir 1 tablespoon Italian seasoning, 2 tablespoons shredded mozzarella or grated Parmesan, and 2 teaspoons tomato paste into the egg yolk mixture.

Nutrition (per serving): 50 calories, 3 g protein, 1 g carbohydrates, 0 g fiber, 0 g sugar, 4 g fat, 2 g saturated fat, 55 mg sodium

EVERYTHING BAGEL CLOUD BREAD: Stir ⅛ teaspoon kosher salt, 1 teaspoon poppy seeds, 1 teaspoon sesame seeds, 1 teaspoon minced dried garlic, and 1 teaspoon minced dried onion (or use 1 tablespoon everything bagel seasoning) into the egg yolk mixture.

Nutrition (per serving): 60 calories, 3 g protein, 1 g carbohydrates, 0 g fiber, 0 g sugar, 4.5 g fat, 2 g saturated fat, 80 mg sodium

RANCH CLOUD BREAD: Stir 1½ teaspoons ranch seasoning powder into the egg yolk mixture.

Nutrition (per serving): 50 calories, 3 g protein, 0 g carbohydrates, 0 g fiber, 0 g sugar, 4 g fat, 2 g saturated fat, 90 mg sodium

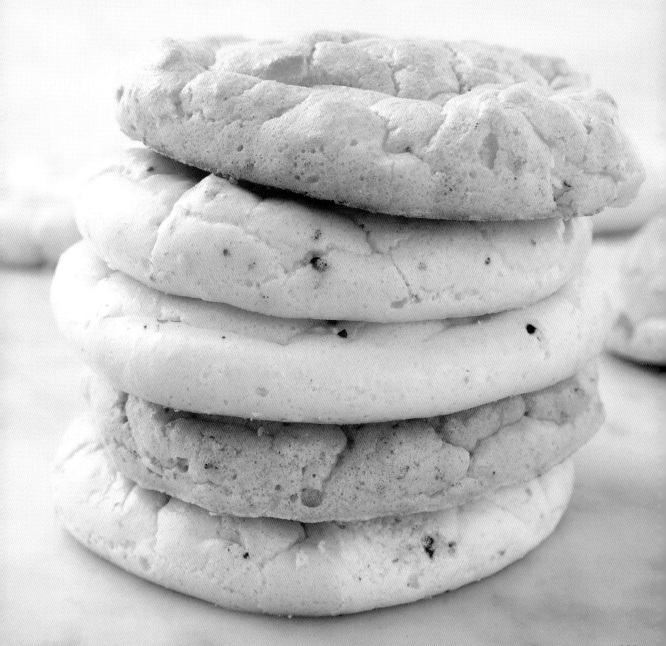

CHEESY CAULI BREAD

TOTAL TIME: 45 MIN / SERVES 6

Essentially a cauliflower crust pizza sliced into breadsticks. Yes, please.

- 1 large head cauliflower
- 2 large eggs
- 2 cloves garlic, minced
- ½ teaspoon dried oregano
- 3 cups shredded mozzarella, divided
- ½ cup grated Parmesan
- Kosher salt
- Freshly ground black pepper
- Pinch of crushed red pepper flakes
- 2 teaspoons freshly chopped parsley
- Marinara sauce, for dipping

1. Preheat oven to 425° and line a baking sheet with parchment paper. On a box grater or in a food processor, grate cauliflower.

2. Transfer cauliflower to a large bowl and add eggs, garlic, oregano, 1 cup mozzarella, and Parmesan, and season with salt and pepper. Stir until completely combined.

3. Transfer dough to prepared baking sheet and pat into a crust. Bake until golden and dried out, 25 minutes.

4. Sprinkle with remaining mozzarella, crushed red pepper flakes, and parsley and bake until cheese is melted, 5 to 10 minutes more.

5. Slice and serve with marinara.

Nutrition (per serving): 230 calories, 20 g protein, 10 g carbohydrates, 7 g fiber, 3 g sugar, 13 g fat, 7 g saturated fat, 430 mg sodium

BROCCOLI CHEESY BREAD

TOTAL TIME: 40 MIN / SERVES 8

If your favorite soup is broccoli cheddar, you better believe you're going to devour a plate of this in one sitting.

- 3 cups riced broccoli
- 1 large egg
- 1½ cups shredded mozzarella, divided
- ¼ cup freshly grated Parmesan
- 2 cloves garlic, minced
- ½ teaspoon dried oregano
- Kosher salt
- Freshly ground black pepper
- 2 teaspoons freshly chopped parsley
- Pinch of crushed red pepper flakes (optional)
- Warmed marinara sauce, for serving

1. Preheat oven to 425° and line a large baking sheet with parchment paper. Microwave riced broccoli for 1 minute to steam. Carefully ring out extra moisture from the broccoli using paper towel or cheese cloth.

2. Transfer broccoli to a large bowl and add egg, 1 cup mozzarella, Parmesan, and garlic. Season with oregano, salt, and pepper. Transfer dough to baking sheet and shape into a thin, round crust.

3. Bake until golden and dried out, 20 minutes. Top with remaining ½ cup mozzarella and bake until cheese is melted and crust is crispy, 10 minutes more.

4. Garnish with parsley and pepper flakes if using. Serve warm with marinara.

Nutrition (per serving): 110 calories, 9 g protein, 6 g carbohydrates, 2 g fiber, 1 g sugar, 6 g fat, 3 g saturated fat, 210 mg sodium

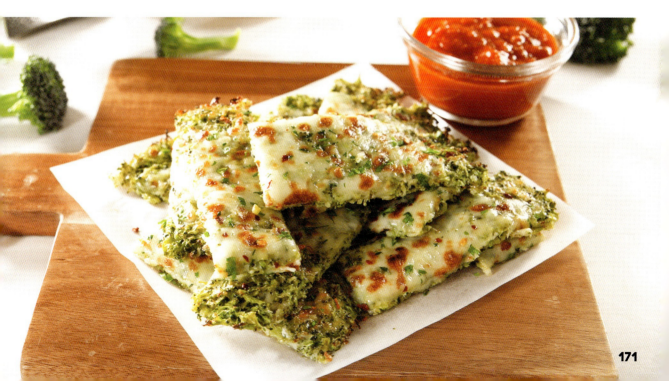

CAULIFLOWER GARLIC BREAD

TOTAL TIME: 1 HR 10 MIN / SERVES 8

Almond flour, eggs, and cauliflower rice are the base of this flavorful low-carb bread.

- 3 cups cauliflower, riced
- 6 large eggs, separated
- 1¼ cups almond flour
- 1 tablespoon baking powder
- 1 teaspoon kosher salt
- 6 tablespoons butter (¾ stick), melted
- 5 cloves garlic, minced
- 1 tablespoon chopped thyme
- 1 tablespoon parsley, chopped, divided
- Parmesan, for serving

1. Preheat oven to 350° and line a 9"-x-5" loaf pan with parchment paper. In a medium bowl, microwave cauliflower for 3 to 4 minutes or until soft and tender. Let cool. When cool enough to handle, transfer cauliflower to a clean kitchen towel and squeeze to release as much moisture as possible.

2. In a medium bowl, beat egg whites until stiff peaks form. Set aside.

3. In a large bowl, whisk together almond flour, baking powder, salt, egg yolks, melted butter, garlic and about ¼ of the whipped egg whites. Beat until well combined, then stir in microwaved cauliflower. Fold in the remaining egg whites and mix until just incorporated. (Mixture should be fluffy.) Fold in the thyme and most of the parsley (save some for topping).

4. Transfer batter to the lined loaf pan and sprinkle with more parsley. Bake until the top is golden, about 45 to 50 minutes. Let cool completely before slicing.

5. Sprinkle slices with Parmesan and more parsley.

Nutrition (per serving): 190 calories, 9 g protein, 7 g carbohydrates, 3 g fiber, 1 g sugar, 15 g fat, 3.5 g saturated fat, 310 mg sodium

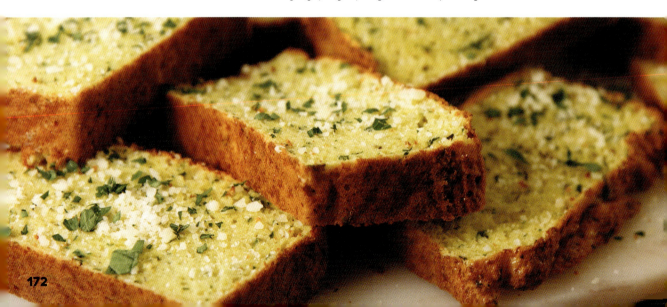

DANGEROUSLY GOOD DESSERTS

Chocolate PB Fat Bombs	175
Magic Cookies	176
Cookie Dough Fat Bombs	179
Coconut Avocado Pops	180
Carrot Cake Balls	180
Peanut Butter Squares	181
Chocolate Truffles	181
Classic Cheesecake	183
Triple Berry Crisp	184
Chocolate Mug Cake	187
Copycat Chocolate Frosty	188
Avocado Brownies	190
Double Chocolate Muffins	191

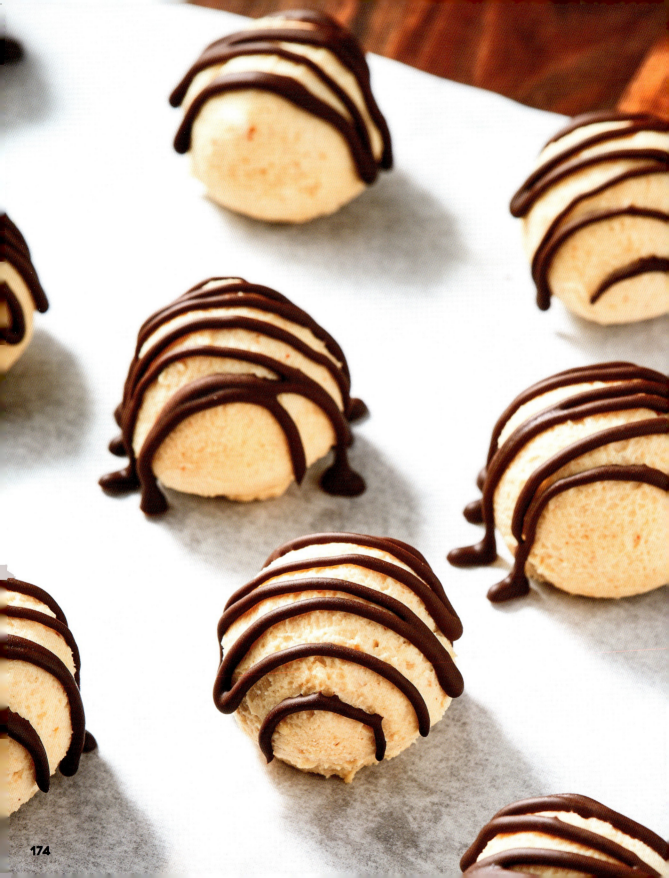

CHOCOLATE PB FAT BOMBS

TOTAL TIME: 25 MIN / SERVES 8

Fat bombs keep you full longer, promote ketosis, and can even increase metabolism. Store them in your fridge and grab a bomb any time you feel your energy waning.

8 ounces cream cheese, softened to room temperature

½ cup keto-friendly peanut butter

¼ cup coconut oil, plus 2 tablespoons

1 teaspoon kosher salt

1 cup keto-friendly dark chocolate chips (such as Lily's)

1. Line a small baking sheet with parchment paper. In a medium bowl, combine cream cheese, peanut butter, ¼ cup coconut oil, and salt. Using a hand mixer, beat mixture until fully combined, about 2 minutes. Place bowl in freezer to firm up slightly, 10 to 15 minutes.

2. When peanut butter mixture has hardened, use a small cookie scoop or spoon to create golf ball–sized balls. Place in the refrigerator to reharden, 5 minutes.

3. Meanwhile, make chocolate drizzle: Combine chocolate chips and remaining coconut oil in a microwave-safe bowl and microwave in 30-second intervals until fully melted. Drizzle over peanut butter balls and place back in the refrigerator to re-harden, another 5 minutes. Serve chilled.

4. To store, keep covered in refrigerator.

Nutrition (per serving): 290 calories, 5 g protein, 5 g carbohydrates, 1 g fiber, 2 g sugar, 28 g fat, 16 g saturated fat, 390 mg sodium

MAGIC COOKIES

TOTAL TIME: 25 MIN / SERVES 18

The most magical part of these cookies? The batter is just coconut oil, butter, and egg yolks. Swap in your favorite nut.

¼ cup coconut oil

4 tablespoons (½ stick) butter, softened

2 tablespoons Swerve sweetener

4 large egg yolks

1 cup sugar-free dark chocolate chips, (such as Lily's)

1 cup unsweetened coconut flakes

¾ cup roughly chopped walnuts

1 Preheat oven to 350° and line a baking sheet with parchment paper. In a large bowl stir together coconut oil, butter, sweetener, and egg yolks. Mix in chocolate chips, coconut, and walnuts.

2 Drop batter by the spoonful onto prepared baking sheet and bake until golden, 15 minutes.

Nutrition (per serving): 130 calories, 2 g protein, 2 g carbohydrates, 1 g fiber, 0 g sugar, 13 g fat, 8 g saturated fat, 25 mg sodium

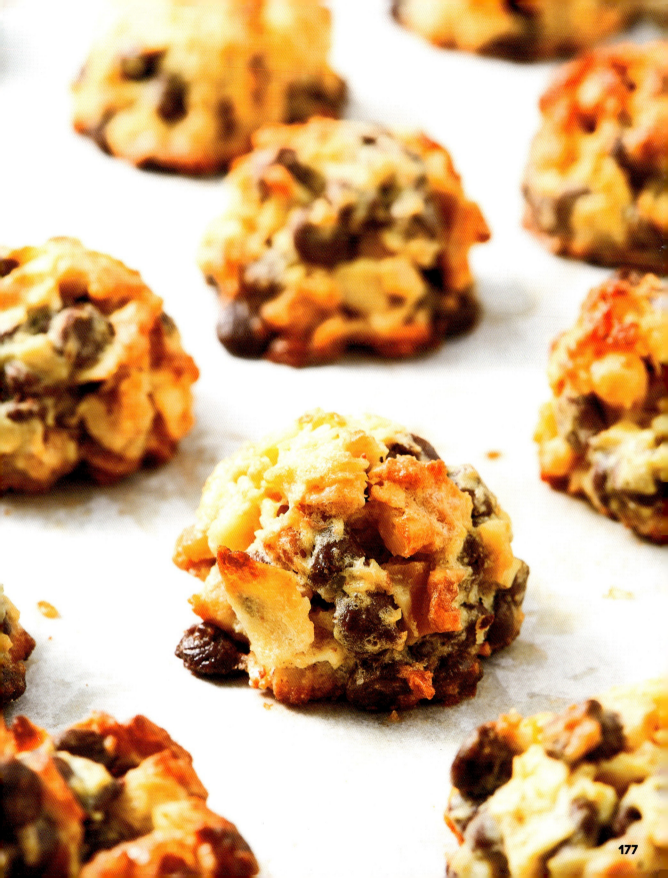

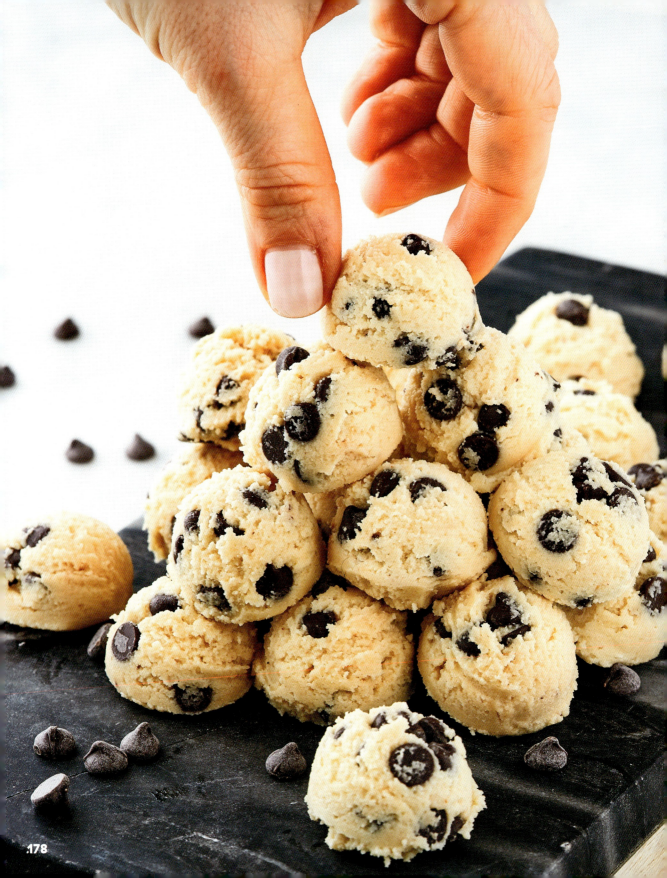

COOKIE DOUGH FAT BOMBS

TOTAL TIME: 1 HR 5 MIN / SERVES 30

Yup, you can eat cookie dough on keto. You just have to swap in a keto-friendly sweetener (Swerve's our fave).

8 tablespoons (1 stick) butter, softened to room temperature

⅓ cup keto-friendly confectioners' sugar (such as Swerve)

½ teaspoon pure vanilla extract

½ teaspoon kosher salt

2 cups almond flour

⅔ cup dark chocolate chips (such as Lily's)

1. In a large bowl using a hand mixer, beat butter until light and fluffy. Add sugar, vanilla, and salt and beat until combined.

2. Slowly beat in your almond flour until no dry spots remain, then fold in chocolate chips. Cover bowl with plastic wrap and place in refrigerator to firm slightly, 15 to 20 minutes.

3. Using a small cookie scoop, scoop dough into small balls. Store in the refrigerator if planning to eat within the week, or in the freezer for up to 1 month.

Nutrition (per serving): 70 calories, 2 g protein, 2 g carbohydrates, 1 g fiber, 0 g sugar, 7 g fat, 2 g saturated fat, 35 mg sodium

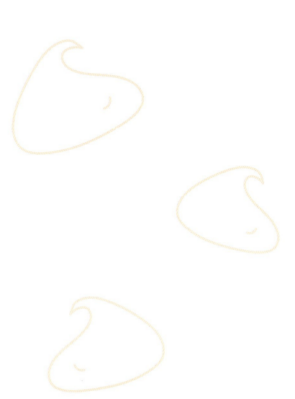

COCONUT AVOCADO POPS

TOTAL TIME: 6 HR 10 MIN / SERVES 10

Avocado might be your favorite fruit for snacking, but it's also amazing in desserts, thanks to its ultra-creamy texture. You're gonna want a batch of these avocado pops in your freezer stat.

- 3 ripe avocados, pitted and peeled
- Juice of 2 limes (about ⅓ cup)
- 3 tablespoons keto-friendly powdered sugar sweetener (such as Swerve)
- ¾ cup coconut milk
- 1 cup keto-friendly chocolate chips (such as Lily's)
- 1 tablespoon coconut oil

1. Into a blender or food processor, combine avocados with lime juice, Swerve, and coconut milk. Blend until smooth and pour into popsicle molds.
2. Freeze until firm, 6 hours up to overnight.
3. In a medium bowl, combine chocolate chips and coconut oil. Microwave on high until melted, then let cool to room temperature. Dunk frozen pops in melted chocolate and serve immediately.

Nutrition (per serving): 120 calories, 1 g protein, 5 g carbohydrates, 3 g fiber, 0 g sugar, 12 g fat, 5 g saturated fat, 5 mg sodium

CARROT CAKE BALLS

TOTAL TIME: 15 MIN / SERVES 16

Everything you love about carrot cake gets transformed into a bite-sized dessert.

- 1 (8-ounce) block cream cheese, softened
- ¾ cup coconut flour
- 1 teaspoon stevia
- ½ teaspoon pure vanilla extract
- 1 teaspoon cinnamon
- ¼ teaspoon ground nutmeg
- 1 cup grated carrots
- ½ cup chopped pecans
- 1 cup shredded unsweetened coconut

1. In a large bowl, using a hand mixer, beat together cream cheese, coconut flour, stevia, vanilla, cinnamon, and nutmeg. Fold in carrots and pecans.
2. Roll into 16 balls then roll in shredded coconut and serve immediately.

Nutrition (per serving): 130 calories, 2 g protein, 6 g carbohydrates, 3 g fiber, 2 g sugar, 11 g fat, 7 g saturated fat, 65 mg sodium

PEANUT BUTTER SQUARES

TOTAL TIME: 2 HR 15 MIN / SERVES 12

These squares taste best cold, so keep them refrigerated until ready to serve.

Cooking spray, for pan

1½ cups smooth unsweetened peanut butter

1¼ cups coconut flour

¼ cup keto-friendly powdered sugar, (such as Swerve)

1 teaspoon pure vanilla extract

Pinch of kosher salt

2 cups keto-friendly chocolate chips, (such as Lily's)

2 tablespoons coconut oil

1 tablespoon flaky sea salt, for garnish

1 Line an 8"-x-8" baking pan with parchment paper and grease with cooking spray. In a medium bowl, combine peanut butter, coconut flour, powdered sugar, vanilla, and salt. Stir until smooth and pour into prepared pan, smoothing the top with a spatula. Place in freezer for 30 minutes to firm up.

2 Combine chocolate chips and coconut oil in a medium microwave-safe bowl. Microwave on high, stirring every 30 seconds, until smooth and pourable. Pour chocolate over peanut butter layer and smooth it.

3 Garnish with flaky sea salt and place in freezer to harden, 2 hours or up to overnight.

4 When ready to serve, remove peanut butter bars from baking dish and cut into squares.

Nutrition (per serving): 280 calories, 9 g protein, 14 g carbohydrates, 6 g fiber, 3 g sugar, 20 g fat, 6 g saturated fat, 540 mg sodium

CHOCOLATE TRUFFLES

TOTAL TIME: 30 MIN / SERVES 15

No diet is complete without chocolate. Store these in your fridge and indulge whenever!

1 cup keto-friendly dark chocolate chips, melted

1 medium avocado, pitted, peeled and smashed

1 teaspoon vanilla extract

¼ teaspoon kosher salt

¼ cup cocoa powder

1 In a medium bowl, combine melted chocolate with avocado, vanilla, and salt. Stir together until smooth and fully combined. Place in the refrigerator to firm up slightly, 15 to 20 minutes.

2 When chocolate mixture has stiffened, use a small cookie scoop or small spoon to scoop approximately 1 tablespoon of the chocolate mixture. Roll chocolate in the palm of your hand until round, then roll in cocoa powder.

Nutrition (per serving): 20 calories, 1 g protein, 2 g carbohydrates, 1 g fiber, 0 g sugar, 2 g fat, 0 g saturated fat, 35 mg sodium

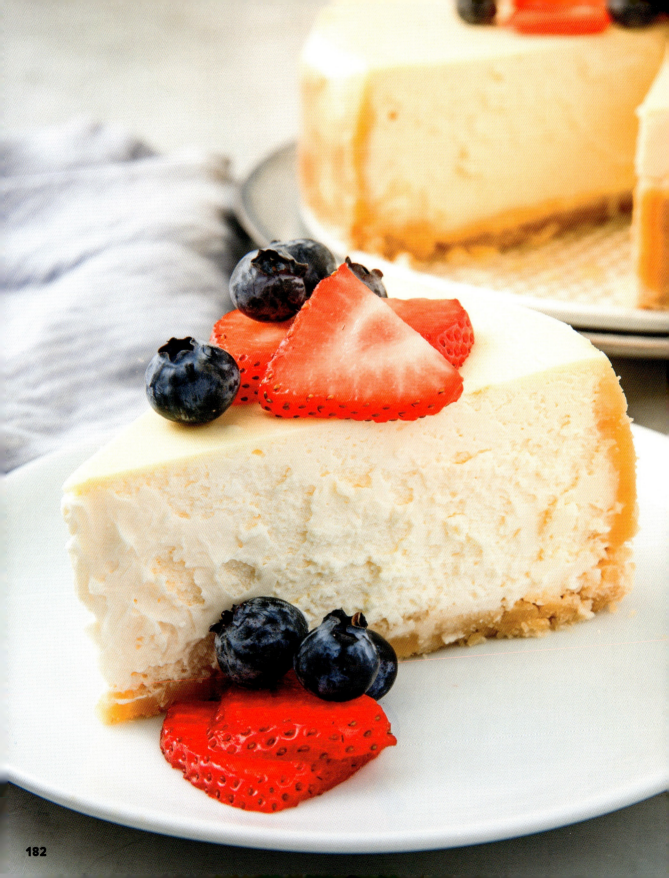

CLASSIC CHEESECAKE

TOTAL TIME: 8 HR / SERVES 8 TO 10

With a crust made of almond and coconut flours, this rich, creamy cheesecake is everything.

Cooking spray, for pan

½ cup almond flour

½ cup coconut flour

¼ cup shredded coconut

½ cup (1 stick) butter, melted

3 (8-ounce) blocks cream cheese, softened to room temperature

16 ounces sour cream, at room temperature

1 tablespoon stevia

2 teaspoons pure vanilla extract

3 large eggs, at room temperature

Sliced strawberries, for serving

1 Preheat oven to 300°. Grease an 8"- or 9"-inch springform pan, and cover the bottom and edges with foil. In a medium bowl, mix together the flours, coconut, and butter. Press the crust into the bottom and a little up the sides of the prepared pan. Place the pan in the fridge while you make the filling.

2 In a large bowl, beat the cream cheese and sour cream together, then beat in the stevia and vanilla. Add the eggs one at a time, mixing after each addition. Spread the filling evenly over the crust.

3 Place pan in a water bath, then bake until it only slightly jiggles in the center, 1 hour to 1 hour 20 minutes. Turn oven off, but leave the cake in the oven with the door slightly ajar to cool slowly for an hour.

4 Remove pan from water bath and take off foil then let chill in the fridge for at least 5 hours or up to overnight. Slice and garnish with strawberries.

Nutrition (per serving): 500 calories, 10 g protein, 10 g carbohydrates, 3 g fiber, 5 g sugar, 47 g fat, 27 g saturated fat, 270 mg sodium

TRIPLE BERRY CRISP

TOTAL TIME: 40 MIN / MAKES 10

This riff on a classic crisp skips blueberries—they're just a little higher in carbs. Top with a spoonful of yogurt for some creaminess.

Cooking spray, for baking dish

1 (6-ounce) package raspberries

1 (6-ounce) package blackberries

1 cup hulled and sliced strawberries

1 teaspoon lemon zest

2 teaspoons lemon juice

1 teaspoon stevia, divided

1 teaspoon vanilla extract

2 tablespoons plus ¾ cup almond flour, divided

¾ cup finely chopped pecans

2 tablespoons ground flax seed

¼ teaspoon cinnamon

3 tablespoons butter, softened

1 Preheat the oven to 350° and grease an 8"-x-8" baking dish with cooking spray. In a large bowl, mix berries, lemon zest, lemon juice, ½ teaspoon stevia, vanilla, and 2 tablespoons almond flour until combined. Spread mixture into bottom of prepared baking dish.

2 In a medium bowl, add remaining ¾ cup almond flour, pecans, flax seed, cinnamon, remaining ½ teaspoon stevia, and butter. Using a fork or clean hands, toss until coarse crumbs form. Sprinkle over berries.

3 Bake until crumble is golden, about 30 to 35 minutes, checking and covering with foil if browning too much. Cool slightly before serving.

Nutrition (per serving): 170 calories, 4 g protein, 9 carbohydrates, 5 g fiber, 3 g sugar, 15 g fat, 3 g saturated fat, 35 mg sodium

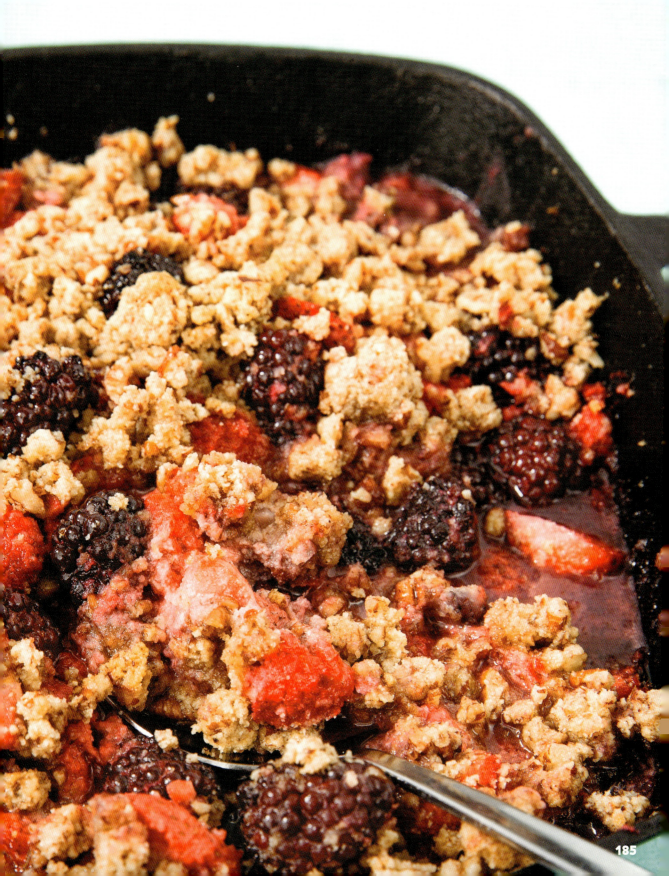

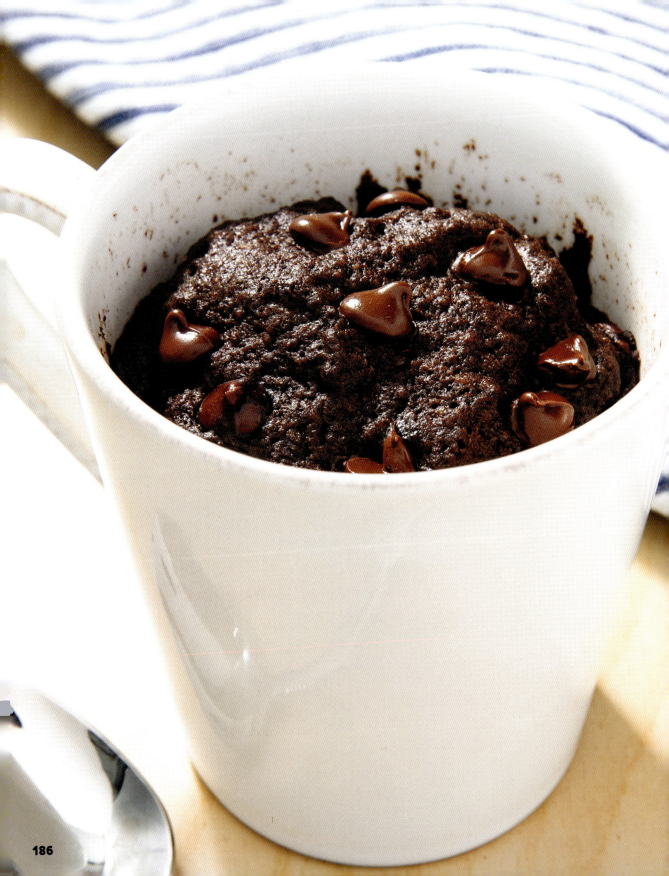

CHOCOLATE MUG CAKE

TOTAL TIME: 5 MIN / SERVES 1

Mug cakes are a big thing on Pinterest, and we can see why: This rich cake takes only five minutes to make from start to finish.

2 tablespoons (¼ stick) butter
¼ cup almond flour
2 tablespoons cocoa powder
1 large egg, beaten
2 tablespoons keto-friendly chocolate chips (such as Lily's)
1 teaspoon Swerve sweetener
½ teaspoon baking powder
Pinch of kosher salt

1 Place butter in a microwave-safe mug and heat until melted, 30 seconds. Add remaining ingredients and stir until fully combined. Cook for 45 seconds to 1 minute, or until cake is set but still fudgy.

Nutrition (per serving): 470 calories, 15 g protein, 13 g carbohydrates, 7 g fiber, 1 g sugar, 44 g fat, 18 g saturated fat, 530 mg sodium

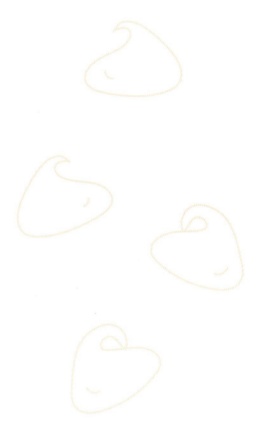

COPYCAT CHOCOLATE FROSTY

TOTAL TIME: 45 MIN / SERVES 4

If you're a sucker for the Wendy's cult favorite, this frosty is surprisingly close to the real thing.

- 1½ cups heavy cream
- 2 tablespoons unsweetened cocoa powder
- 3 tablespoons keto-friendly powdered sugar sweetener (such as Swerve)
- 1 teaspoon pure vanilla extract
- Pinch of kosher salt

1. In a large bowl, combine cream, cocoa, sweetener, vanilla, and salt. Using a hand mixer or the whisk attachment of a stand mixer, beat mixture until stiff peaks form. Scoop mixture into a plastic zip-top bag and freeze 30 to 35 minutes, until just frozen.

2. Cut tip off zip-top bag and pipe into serving dishes.

Nutrition (per serving): 320 calories, 2 g protein, 4 g carbohydrates, 1 g fiber, 0 g sugar, 34 g fat, 21 g saturated fat, 35 mg sodium

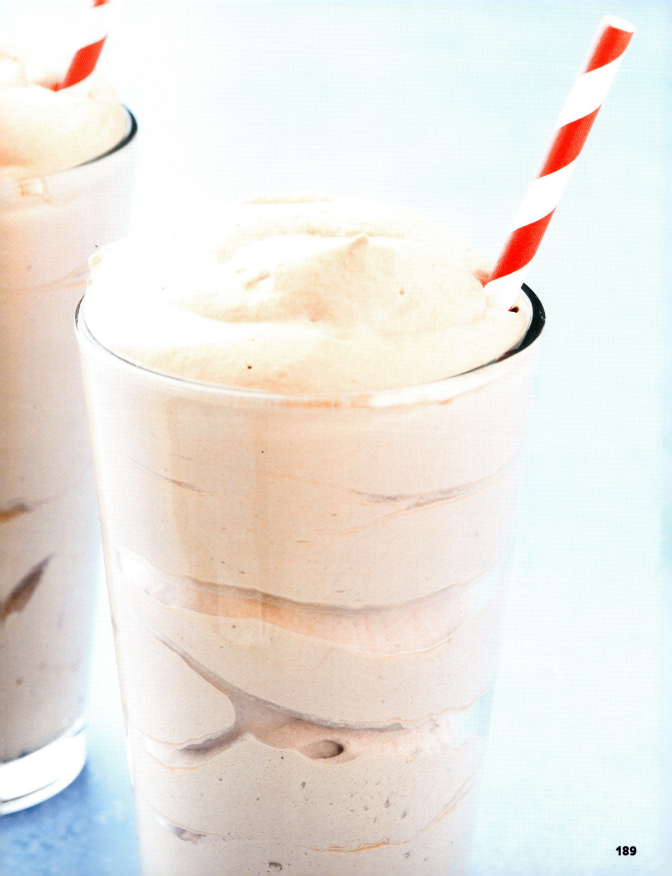

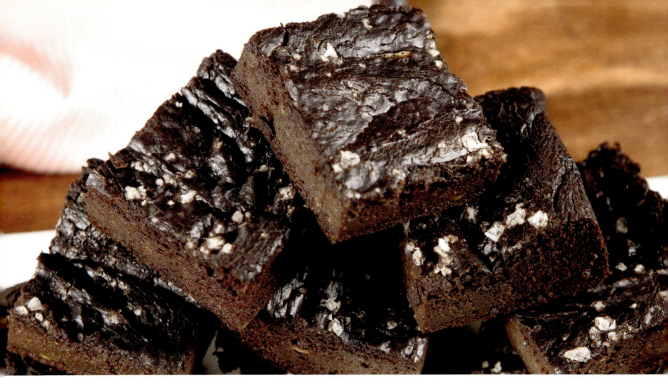

AVOCADO BROWNIES

TOTAL TIME: 1 HR 25 MIN / SERVES 16

When the chocolate craving is real, these brownies hit the spot.

4 large eggs

2 ripe avocados, pitted and peeled

½ cup (1 stick) melted butter

6 tablespoons unsweetened peanut butter

2 teaspoons baking soda

⅔ cup keto-friendly granulated sugar (such as Swerve)

⅔ cup unsweetened cocoa powder

2 teaspoons pure vanilla extract

½ teaspoon kosher salt

Flaky sea salt (optional)

1 Preheat oven to 350° and line an 8"-x-8" square pan with parchment paper. In a blender or food processor, combine all ingredients except flaky sea salt and blend until smooth.

2 Transfer batter to prepared baking pan and smooth the top with a spatula. Top with flaky sea salt, if using.

3 Bake until brownies are soft but not at all wet to the touch, 25 to 30 minutes.

4 Let cool 25 to 30 minutes before slicing and serving.

Nutrition (per serving): 160 calories, 4 g protein, 16 g carbohydrates, 5 g fiber, 1 g sugar, 14 g fat, 5 g saturated fat, 283 mg sodium

DOUBLE CHOCOLATE MUFFINS

TOTAL TIME: 25 MIN / SERVES 12

They might be called muffins, but they'll fool anyone into thinking they're cupcakes.

- 2 cups almond flour
- ¾ cup unsweetened cocoa powder
- ¼ cup keto-friendly powdered sugar, (such as Swerve)
- 1½ teaspoons baking powder
- 1 teaspoon kosher salt
- 1 cup (2 sticks) butter, melted
- 3 large eggs
- 1 teaspoon pure vanilla extract
- 1 cup sugar-free dark chocolate chips (such as Lily's)

1. Preheat oven to 350° and line a muffin tin with paper liners. In a large bowl whisk together almond flour, cocoa powder, Swerve, baking powder, and salt. Add melted butter, eggs, and vanilla and stir until combined.

2. Fold in chocolate chips.

3. Divide batter among muffin liners and bake until a toothpick inserted into the middle comes out clean, 12 minutes.

Nutrition (per serving): 280 calories, 7 g protein, 7 g carbohydrates, 4 g fiber, 1 g sugar, 27 g fat, 11 g saturated fat, 90 mg sodium

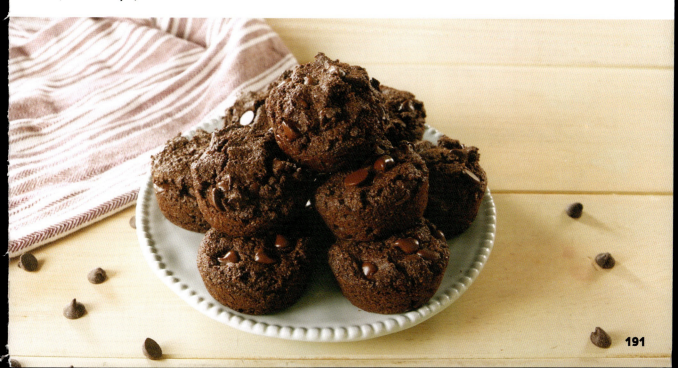

ADD TO YOUR DELISH COLLECTION

You'll find everything you could possibly want in one of our cookbooks—whether it's a weeknight chicken dinner, an easy Instant Pot side, an epic air fryer appetizer, or an over-the-top dessert. We've got it all.

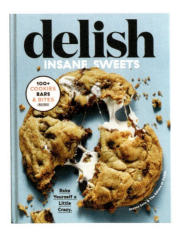

INSANE SWEETS
100+ Cookies, Bars, Bites & Treats

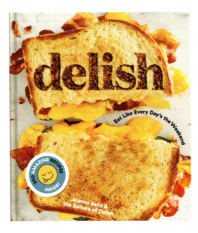

EAT LIKE EVERY DAY'S THE WEEKEND
275+ Recipes Made To Be Devoured

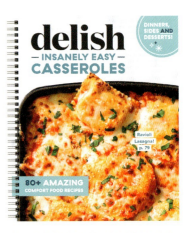

INSANELY EASY CASSEROLES
80+ Amazing Comfort Food Recipes

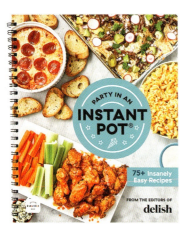

PARTY IN AN INSTANT POT
75+ Fun Dishes To Make In Your Multi Cooker

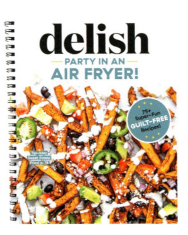

PARTY IN AN AIR FRYER
75+ Super-Fun, Guilt-Free Recipes

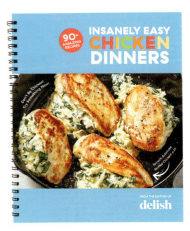

INSANELY EASY CHICKEN DINNERS
90+ Delicious Dinners

CHECK THEM OUT AT: Store.Delish.com or Amazon.com.